Physical Education Assessment Toolkit

LIZ GILES-BROWN

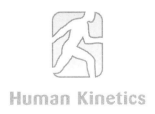

Human Kinetics

Giles-Brown, Elizabeth, 1965-
   Physical education assessment toolkit / Elizabeth Giles-Brown.
      p. cm.
  ISBN 0-7360-5796-X (soft cover)
  1. Physical fitness for children--Testing. 2. Physical education and
training--Study and teaching. I. Title.
  GV436.5.G55 2006
  613.7'042--dc22

                        2005031482

ISBN-10: 0-7360-5796-X
ISBN-13: 978-0-7360-5796-7

The Web addresses cited in this text were current as of December 2005, unless otherwise noted.

Acquisitions Editor: Bonnie Pettifor; **Developmental Editor:** Ray Vallese; **Assistant Editors:** Derek Campbell and Bethany J. Bentley; **Copyeditor:** Bob Replinger; **Proofreader:** Erin Cler; **Permission Manager:** Dalene Reeder; **Graphic Designer:** Bob Reuther; **Graphic Artist:** Dawn Sills; **Photo Manager:** Sarah Ritz; **Cover Designer:** Keith Blomberg; **Photographers (cover):** Sarah Ritz, Tom Roberts, and ©Eyewire/Photodisc/Getty Images; **Photographer (interior):** © Human Kinetics, except where otherwise noted. Photos on pages 155 and 175 by Sarah Ritz; photo on page 121 © Eyewire/Photodisc/Getty Images; **Art Manager:** Kelly Hendren; **Illustrator:** Keri Evans; **Printer:** United Graphics

Printed in the United States of America   10   9   8   7   6   5   4   3   2   1

Human Kinetics
Web site: www.HumanKinetics.com

United States: Human Kinetics
P.O. Box 5076
Champaign, IL 61825-5076
800-747-4457
e-mail: humank@hkusa.com

Canada: Human Kinetics
475 Devonshire Road Unit 100
Windsor, ON N8Y 2L5
800-465-7301 (in Canada only)
e-mail: orders@hkcanada.com

Europe: Human Kinetics
107 Bradford Road
Stanningley
Leeds LS28 6AT, United Kingdom
+44 (0) 113 255 5665
e-mail: hk@hkeurope.com

Australia: Human Kinetics
57A Price Avenue
Lower Mitcham, South Australia 5062
08 8277 1555
e-mail: liaw@hkaustralia.com

New Zealand: Human Kinetics
Division of Sports Distributors NZ Ltd.
P.O. Box 300 226 Albany
North Shore City
Auckland
0064 9 448 1207
e-mail: info@humankinetics.co.nz

Contents

PART II　Model Units and Ideas on Backward Design　205

Consider the thought of having ready-to-use assessments at your fingertips for any unit or lesson you are teaching. Wouldn't it be terrific to have a resource to turn to anytime you need an assessment? Well, here it is! The main goal of *Physical Education Assessment Toolkit* is to provide you with meaningful yet practical ways to assess learning in your classes. All the assessments were designed with today's busy teachers in mind. Just by filling in a reproducible form, included in the book as well as on the accompanying CD-ROM, you can customize an assessment for virtually any unit in physical education. The *Toolkit* also contains three sample units based on the backward design model of unit development that many of our colleagues are implementing in other subject areas. All the units, lessons, and teaching suggestions reflect effective teaching practices as well as current brain-compatible learning principles. The tried-and-true activities included in the lessons have been used successfully with living, breathing children. You can use the units as a guide while planning for quality assessment and as a reference for developing more units for any subject in physical education.

The goal of a quality physical education program is to help children become self-confident movers, gaining the skills, knowledge, and understanding that will motivate them to lead healthy and active lifestyles. Part of achieving that goal is teaching and assessing skill development, but another key is to support that skill development by delving beneath the surface to teach and assess for understanding. If students truly understand the underlying concepts and principles of motor skill development, health- and skill-related fitness, and positive social interactions, ultimately they will develop better skills and be able to make applications in related situations. Teachers must do more than discover what students know and can do. And it's not enough for physical educators to narrow their focus to just getting kids moving for a designated period. To foster the motivation necessary to maintain a healthy and active lifestyle, teachers can use effective assessment to help students become consciously aware of what they can do, what they know, and what they understand.

Many assessment resource books are available to physical education teachers, so why should you choose this one? What makes the *Toolkit* unique? First, each assessment template is reproducible so that you can use it with any unit in an established curriculum or with new unit designs. With this system, you and your students become familiar with the process and thus require less organizational and instructional time each time you use an assessment. Good assessment is part of good teaching, and assessment can be fun and motivating for students and teachers when used in a positive way. A second unique aspect of the *Toolkit* is that it targets a wide range of students. Although the assessments were designed for students in grades three through eight, they could easily be used with high school students with an expectation of more sophisticated responses and more varied skills.

Physical Education Assessment Toolkit consists of this book and a bound-in CD-ROM that together offer 134 assessment forms and nine content-specific posters. Overall, the *Toolkit* provides you with the following:

Part I: Chapters 1 through 9

- Information on how the book is organized and how to use it efficiently
- Valuable teaching tips to help you use time more efficiently and set up students for success
- Ways in which to implement all the assessments, which are also available on the CD-ROM for easy reproduction
- Sample lesson ideas for each type of assessment approach

Part II: Chapters 10 through 12

- Information on how to design units using the backward design model of curriculum development

- Three complete model units that incorporate a variety of the assessments found in the book and on the CD-ROM

Appendix

- An appendix containing guidance for scoring the assessments

CD-ROM

- All the assessment forms from the book in separate PDF files for easy printing and reproduction (See page 280 for details on using the CD-ROM.)
- Half-page forms doubled up in the PDF files for convenience (For example, page 83 of the text features forms 4.18 and 4.19, but the respective PDF files on the CD-ROM contain two copies of each form.)

- Nine color posters that can be printed on letter-size paper or on larger paper, to a maximum size of 25.5 inches by 33 inches
- Support for each of the assessment approaches found in the *Toolkit*
- Content-driven pictures designed for the physical education learning space
- Vocabulary-building terms to support learning and memory

The *Toolkit* will become invaluable for physical educators interested in planning for assessment and taking a backward look at how they design units in their mission of providing their students with lasting skill and knowledge. This resource offers meaningful assessments aimed at the heart of the discipline for teachers who want to help children discover how to apply their knowledge for increased skill development.

PART I

Assessments and Ideas for Implementation

The goal of part I is to provide you with 134 assessment templates that can help students become more self-confident movers, gaining the skills, knowledge, and understanding that will motivate them to lead healthy and active lifestyles. Although this part of the book is dedicated to physical education assessments, good assessment in any discipline cannot stand alone. Good assessment is part of good teaching. It is not enough to organize a variety of assessments without thinking about how to incorporate them into the curriculum.

Chapter 1 will help you understand how the chapters are set up, the format of the templates, how to use the rubrics, the threads in physical education, and the importance of interactions, fitness routines, feedback, the power of choice, music, and modeling. Careful reading of chapter 1 will make it easier to use the rest of the resource. All 134 assessment templates are provided in chapters 2 through 12 and on the accompanying CD-ROM, which also contains 9 content-specific posters. Information and lesson ideas support the assessments and make them easier to use. After reading these chapters and becoming familiar with the assessments, implementing them becomes as easy as printing the forms from the accompanying CD-ROM, filling in the content that you are teaching, and copying them for your students to use. So let's get started.

1
CHAPTER

Using This Resource

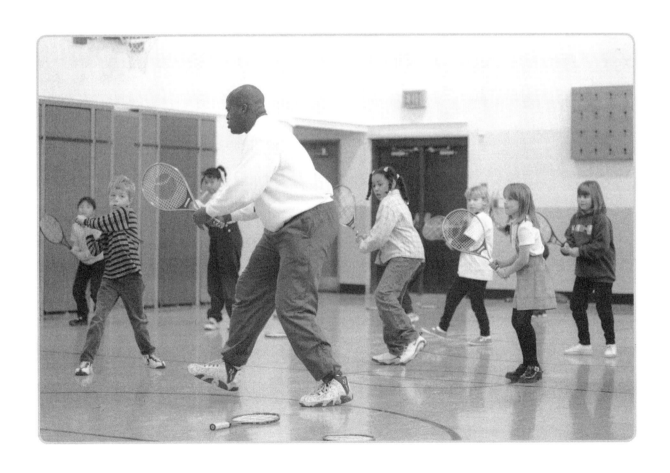

Chapters 2 through 9 all follow the same format. They contain assessments that cover the areas of daily assessment, goal setting and reflecting, motor skills, movement concepts, health- and skill-related fitness, strategy, decorating with content, and closure. Each chapter begins with a brief overview followed by an in-depth explanation of the idea and the assessments. The "Setting Up Everyone for Success" section outlines specific strategies that will help you be more successful when using the ideas and assessments. Next, a chapter summary is followed by

- one or more "Putting It Into Practice" sections that provide ideas on how to implement the assessments;
- one or more lessons or activities that put the assessments to use; and
- all the assessment forms from the chapter. These templates fall into the following categories: written assessments, self-assessment, peer assessment, application or performance assessments, and observational tools. (Chapter 8's color posters appear only on the CD-ROM.)

Part II contains chapters 10 through 12, which are organized into units of instruction and have their own format.

Assessment Template Format

The assessments found in this resource and on the CD-ROM are all in template format. The main advantage of the template format is that you can apply assessments across a range of situations and skills. As a result, this book will be useful in many ways:

- Individual teachers can explore different ways in which to assess their students.
- Teachers in a school district can perform common assessments.
- At the college level, students can learn to develop units with assessments.
- The book can be a useful resource in the professional library of a school or district.

By adding different content, the assessments can be used more than once with the same group of students. If an assessment is effective, produces the desired information from students, is easy for students to understand, and does not take a large amount of instructional time to implement, why

not use it more than once? When an assessment is found to be effective and students become accustomed to the format, the quality of their work will improve, becoming more specific and detailed. Students have a chance to improve their performance by having more than one trial.

An additional benefit of the template format is that the assessments can be used at more than one level of instruction, with a wide range of students. Although the assessments are intended for grades three through eight, many can be used with high school students with an expectation of more sophisticated responses. These assessment templates can be incorporated into a system of assessment that over time becomes easy for you to organize and implement. This system will yield good information about what students can do, what they know, and what they understand.

Scoring With Rubrics

Scoring student work is sometimes difficult. If a concrete scoring guide is not in place, a number or letter grade attached to an assessment often has little meaning and doesn't tell the student anything specific about his or her performance. An explicit scoring guide is perhaps the most important part of helping students see the target. When students know and understand exactly what they are shooting for, the number of times that they will hit their target will increase. Scoring student work is much easier and more enjoyable when students understand what is being asked.

When students don't understand what is being asked, teachers often blame them for not paying attention. Let's look at this from a different perspective. If the directions are vague or given in a way that is difficult to understand, a large number of students may do poorly. If this occurs, you should look at your instructional practices or the assessment itself.

A scoring rubric accompanies most of the assessments in this resource. The rubrics spell out in qualitative terms what students need to include in a response to receive a specific score. More important, the rubrics appear right along with the directions for the assessment. Why shouldn't students know exactly how their work is to be scored? If students learn how to use the scoring rubric to assess their own work before handing it in or performing their skills, they will hit their target more often. Suddenly, scoring their work becomes more enjoyable and efficient.

The scores on the templates use a four-point scale with a description of what each number represents.

- The highest score of 4 represents excellent work that exceeds the standard. The descriptor indicates just what a student needs to do to earn that score.
- Meeting the standard earns a score of 3, which often means that the work is complete and correct with nothing missing.
- A score of 2 indicates that the student made an attempt but that a few things are missing or incomplete.
- A score of 1 indicates that the student did not understand the assessment, did not put much effort into it, or does not possess the knowledge, skills, or understanding to complete it successfully.

This type of scoring system can easily be integrated into a traditional grading system by assigning letter grades to the numbers. For example, a score of 4 might be equivalent to an A and a score of 3 might be a B. This scoring system is adaptable to many systems already in place.

Threads of Physical Education

This resource also focuses on specific strategies that you can use to set the stage for more learning to occur and ways in which you can thread throughout the curriculum elements common to most physical education classes and physical activity settings. These strategies and threads revolve around the themes of interactions, consensus decision making, conflict resolution, fitness routines, feedback, the power of choice, music, and modeling. Included in this chapter are organizational strategies to help you and your students use time more efficiently as well as ways in which you can induce kids to take responsibility for their learning, attitudes, actions, and interactions. Some of these strategies may take a little time to implement, but over the long haul they will save time that is often used to deal with transitions, off-task behavior, disagreements, and routine conflicts. The strategies also provide ways to reinforce underlying concepts and thus promote learning in each unit. The ideas will be referred to again in the units found in chapters 10 through 12 as well as in the lesson ideas found in chapters that focus on specific types of assessment.

Interactions

Students need to be able to work with all others in the class without doing damage to anyone physically or emotionally. You can easily spot someone who is hurting others physically, but in a busy physical education class you may be unable to pick up emotional damage that can happen in subtle ways. The simple act of asking students to choose partners can be wonderful for some students but devastating for others. Watching a student stand there while others run by, getting who they want for a partner and being sure not to be with the less skilled or less popular students, can be heartbreaking. Students can be taught to practice the virtues that make them better people. The feelings that students have when participating in your class are tied to you and physical activity. Many of us have heard adults talk about bad experiences that they had in school. They remember them because they are embedded in their emotional memory. Emotional memories, positive and negative, stay with us forever.

If we as physical education professionals want to help children develop the skills and knowledge they need to lead healthy and active lives, then we had better pay attention to the emotions that they experience in our classes. Taking time to help them learn about virtues, body language, objectivity, and how to celebrate each other's differences can have a profound effect on how classes run and the feelings that each student associates with physical activity.

Practicing Virtues By identifying the virtues (honesty, self-discipline, or whatever you want to focus on during any lesson or unit) that students need to practice to improve their interactions, you can help them have positive experiences during class. Taking a few seconds to refer to a virtue during a class can have a powerful effect on how students interact. Doing this sets them up to succeed in meeting your expectations. By asking students to identify the virtues that they should practice to increase the chances of success during different activities, you can stress their importance and make students more aware of them.

For example, if a boundary rule in an activity requires students to make a judgment themselves on whether they went out of bounds, you might ask the question, "What virtue is important to practice when thinking about the boundary rule in this activity?" The desired response might be honesty or self-discipline. Having them make that identification is more effective than just giving them the answer. By taking time to do this regularly, you help students build and use the vocabulary, and practice the behaviors that go along with it. The virtues included in some of the self-assessments in this book are respect, responsibility, perseverance, self-discipline, honesty, compassion, courage, and trustworthiness.

Body Language   Students need to be aware of the ways in which people communicate. They need to know that they can send clear verbal messages to others but that they also send clear nonverbal messages, some of which can be hurtful. When you assign two students to work together and one student is unhappy with the assignment, that unhappiness is often evident in body language and facial expressions. The message is often unmistakable and can be hurtful to the student on the receiving end. Having students partner up has always been a practice of physical educators, and they have done it in many different ways. The partnering process puts students in a vulnerable situation. Whether you put students in partnerships or ask students to find partners themselves, you need to teach them how to do it in a positive way. You also need to teach them what kind of effect their body language can have in this situation.

A role play is an excellent way to get this message across, and students will enjoy your participation. As students are learning the procedure for getting partners, have them sit down for a moment. Ask a few students to participate in a role play about getting partners. When you have your volunteers, ask one of the volunteers to be the teacher and have that student ask you and the other volunteer to be partners. Here you can use your acting skills to demonstrate negative body language. Do the role play a few times, communicating different messages through nonverbal communication each time. Use the following discussion questions to help students discover the power of body language.

- What message did I communicate to my assigned partner?
- How do you suppose that made her or him feel?
- Do you think that he or she would feel like working hard after receiving a message like that?

- Do we want people to feel good or bad about themselves when they are in physical education class?
- What can we do to help people feel good about themselves? Why is that important?

Objectivity   This book contains several assessments that involve peers armed with specific criteria playing the role of assessor. Throwing students into that role without guidance about objectivity can set up both those doing the assessment and those being assessed for failure. Not all students know what it means to be objective. Even those who know what it means may have difficulty practicing it. Students need to be taught to look at the movement itself and detach it from the person. The ideal is to reach the point where students doing peer assessment don't care whether they are assessing their best friend or someone with whom they are not friendly.

As with the subject of body language, performing a role play with your students can be effective. Include some talk about virtues in this learning situation. You can take the role of someone who has as a partner his or her best friend, with the friend's performance not meeting the criteria for the highest score. Another scenario would be to take the role of being partnered with someone who is not a good friend, maybe someone with whom there is sometimes enmity, and have the partner's performance be flawless. Here are some discussion questions to use after the acting is over.

- What does it mean to be objective?
- What does it mean to be subjective?
- Do you feel that I was able to be objective in the role play?
- What might have made it hard for me to be objective?
- How is being honest related to being objective?
- How is self-discipline related to being objective?
- What other virtues do you have to practice when trying to be objective?
- How could subjectivity interfere with learning?

Celebrating Differences   Children in our schools are different from one another in many ways. Some are great at writing, math, or reading, whereas some struggle. Some children can run, throw, and kick with ease. Others have a difficult time learning those skills. Throughout a child's years in school we as educators often fail to address how children can celebrate these differences instead of thinking of them in a negative way.

The three differences that stick out in physical education settings are fitness level, skill level, and physical size. Society as a whole places a high value on these traits, and the children in our schools reflect society. These differences between students are right out there for everyone to see, especially in physical education. Students need to participate in lessons and discussions about how to deal with the differences among them in a positive way. They need to be confronted with the damage that they can do to others by drawing attention to differences in a negative way.

Students need to learn that when working in groups or with partners they will sometimes be more skilled, sometimes be equally matched, and sometimes be not as skilled. They also need to know that being in any of these situations is OK and that they have the power to behave in a way that makes it a positive learning experience for everyone. Although the student's job in each situation will be different, everyone can learn. Discussing these roles periodically throughout the year will help students make positive decisions in dealing with the differences among them.

Consensus Decision Making   One of the age-old goals of physical education teachers is to have students who are able to cooperate with each other to work toward group goals. Think about this: Do all students have a clear picture of what cooperation is? Do they know what it takes to cooperate with others, even when they aren't best buddies? When we put kids into groups and expect everything to go smoothly without letting them practice the process of consensus decision making and conflict resolution, we set up students to fail and set up ourselves for disappointment.

The process of consensus decision making is simple and is regularly used in education and business. Good leaders know that a group who participates in making a decision is more likely to support it. We can apply the same kind of thinking to physical education classes. All of our cooperative and competitive activities require getting a group of people to agree to follow a plan. Who gets to come up with the plan? Students need to use the process chosen for decision making repeatedly so

that they get really good at it. It's like any other skill: The more they practice correctly, the better they will get.

The following process can be used with partners or groups depending on the level of the students. Begin by using it with partners in primary grades for simple decisions. When the process becomes a natural thing to do, students can move on to using it in small groups. To use this process successfully in physical education classes, students need to know the difference between giving orders and making polite requests. Students can practice the following steps first by doing role plays and then by using them during the course of a lesson.

Consensus Decision-Making Process

1. Partners or group members sit facing each other.

2. Each person gets a chance to share ideas.

3. The group then uses thumbs to show their preference for the ideas. Thumbs up means, "Yeah! This is my favorite idea!" Thumbs sideways means, "It's not my favorite idea, but I will support it and give my best effort." Thumbs down means, "I can't support this idea or plan."

4. If a person votes thumbs down, he or she must have a good reason. Voting thumbs down in order to sabotage is not permissible.

No one in the group is permitted to take charge and give orders to other group members. Like throwing, catching, and kicking, consensus decision-making is a skill that students must practice.

Conflict Resolution

Conflict resolution is sometimes difficult for adults, let alone children. Many times, students are taught a conflict resolution process, participate in a few role plays, and then are expected to be good at resolving their conflicts all the time. Kids need help practicing the skill of resolving conflicts in real-life situations. What might seem to us like inconsequential conflicts are sometimes important to a child, and we should not ignore them.

To gain competence at these skills, students need to practice respectful listening, making polite requests instead of giving orders, and making "I" statements. An "I" statement is a way of expressing feelings without blaming others for them. Instead of saying, "You cheated and you make me mad when you do that," the person might say, "I get upset when people don't follow the rules. It's frustrating. I would like it if you would follow the rules so that the game is fun for everyone." With a strong process of conflict resolution in place you won't have to spend time trying to find the underlying cause of every argument. Children need to learn that conflict is a natural part of being with other people and that most of the time the conflict is not what causes the problem. How the conflict is handled is usually the problem. Modeling respectful ways in which to resolve conflict is crucial. How can educators expect students to be able to resolve conflicts respectfully if we raise our voices to them when they do something that we don't like? If we want students to be able to make polite requests of each other, we must model that in the handling of daily disappointments and snags in lesson plans.

The following process can be taught to every student, starting in kindergarten. Implementation is simple. Begin by designating a space in which students should resolve minor conflicts. In that space place a "talking" object—a beanbag, stuffed animal, or almost anything small. The object is used to designate the first speaker engaged in conflict resolution. Students can be taught the process of conflict resolution in role plays and then use it during class when conflicts arise. If a student forgets and runs to you with a minor conflict, you should gently remind the student that he or she needs to use conflict resolution skills. At times when students forget they will run to you and say something like, "John just. . . ." To reinforce and help students practice this important life skill, respond by asking, "Who is your conflict with?" or "How do we practice resolving conflicts in this class?" The following steps outline the process that students can learn to follow when any minor conflict arises.

1. If somebody does something that you do not like or think is unfair, you need to make a polite request and ask him or her to stop, explaining how what he or she is doing makes you feel.

2. If the person does not listen and refuses to respect your request, then it is your responsibility to take the person into conflict resolution.

3. Politely ask the person to come and talk with you. You both step out of the problem and into the solution by moving to the space in the gym designed for conflict resolution.

4. The person initiating the resolution begins by picking up the object designated for resolution and talks respectfully to the other student using "I" statements and a soft, calm voice instead of a loud, angry voice. When this student is finished, he or she then hands the object to the other student and that student has an opportunity to respond. They converse until they come to consensus on a solution.

5. After they have come to consensus, both students are able to go back into the activity.

6. If either student has difficulty at any time during this process, he or she may ask for help. They need to try it themselves first, but if they need help they just say, "Could you please help us resolve this conflict?"

Students can use this process all the time. After giving the initial directions for an activity, remind students about the process by asking, "How do we resolve conflicts in this class?" When giving directions for group activities, you can also ask students how they will be able to practice honesty (or any other virtue necessary for successful participation) during the activity. When they provide the answer, they own it and are more likely to remember it and practice it.

Fitness Routines

Having established routines helps classes be more organized and flow more naturally. Too many routines will make classes boring. Too many surprises will make classes confusing. Physical education classes can be balanced with routines that serve a purpose and novel approaches that keep kids excited. A major focus of many physical education programs is health- and skill-related physical fitness. But many programs do not allot sufficient time to that goal to have a major effect on fitness levels. Fitness routines developed in class can be designed so that they can be used by students on their own outside class or shared with classroom teachers so that students can participate in them regularly. Another benefit to having fitness routines in place is that students can perform them on demand and sometimes, depending on what the routine entails, listen to directions for the next activity at the same time. This approach allows you to use class time more efficiently. Flexibility, balance, and muscular endurance routines are just a few ways in which you can include health- or skill-related fitness in any unit. You may choose to quiz students periodically on the benefits of each fitness routine.

Feedback

Without efficient use of feedback, only the innately self-directed learners will improve their skills. Feedback is common to all learning and is worth spending some time thinking about. It's always exciting to watch students who naturally reflect on the available feedback and change their movement based on the information to improve. They are the self-directed learners. Not all students do this naturally. They need to be taught to do so. Students need to learn where to get feedback and how they can use it to improve performance. They need to know that the feedback they get from the outcome of their movement should help them improve performance. In addition, they need to know about the different types of feedback so that when they are on the receiving end, they know what to do with it. When they are required to give feedback, they must know the most effective type to use. They need to know the difference between positive, negative, and instructional feedback as well as the characteristics of general and specific feedback. After initial instruction, whenever you require students to give feedback, remind them of the different types and give them a chance to practice.

Power of Choice

Choice is a powerful tool. As an adult, we know that having choices is important. Giving students a choice, even for what may seem inconsequential, gives them a feeling of power and can affect their attitude toward the tasks. For instance, if students have a routine at the end of class when they need to do several things before they leave, give them the choice of what they would like to do first. Some students might choose to get drinks first, whereas others would rather pick up their equipment. If in the end everything gets done in an orderly manner, giving up a little control is worthwhile. In many situations in physical education you can offer students a choice. One way is how they are assessed. Some assessments in this book ask for the same information but in different ways. For example, in chapter 4 several written assessments require students to provide skill cues for a motor skill. Some are straightforward, and some allow students to be creative. Some students love to take the creative route, whereas others prefer to list the answers. Why not give them a choice? This approach will take the focus off the fact that they have an assessment to complete and instead put it on the fact that they get to choose which type of assessment they would like to do.

Music

Music livens up a physical education class. You can use music as a signal that is much friendlier than a loud whistle. When used purposefully, music can cut down on off-task behavior and aid in using time more efficiently. Sometimes you may choose particular music only because the kids love it. At other times you may use music that can have a specific effect on behavior, motivation, and energy level.

Having always known the effect of music on the energy levels and motivation of a class, one year I wanted to learn exactly how much it mattered. Traditionally, my fifth- and sixth-grade students do their mile-run fitness test on the field. Eight times around the field was equal to 1 mile (1.6 kilometers). The year we moved into our new gym, which was much larger than the old one, we had a lot of rain and did most of our practicing inside with music. Students were doing a great job practicing at pacing themselves. When the time came for the mile fitness test, we had a beautiful spring day so we set up outside. Kids who had been able to pace themselves and jog for eight or nine minutes were doing a lot of walking.

Although many variables were involved, I decided to focus on the absence of music. I asked if any students would be interested in doing the test again inside to see if having music on would have any effect on their time. All but one decided that they would like to try. Of course, this experiment was by no means scientific, but every student cut his or her time, some by a considerable margin.

After attending a six-day training by Eric Jensen called Teaching With the Brain in Mind, I discovered many other powers that music can have. I recommend Jensen's work in the area of brain-compatible learning to anyone interested in looking further into the use of music in education.

Modeling

Nothing is more frustrating than hearing a teacher yell at a class in the name of discipline. What is clearly being taught in this situation is that when people do something to upset you, you yell at them. In this situation some sort of conflict has obviously occurred between members of the class and the teacher. Consider this question: How can a teacher expect students to practice conflict resolution skills when he or she is not willing to model it? If physical educators want their students to make fitness and activity a habit, shouldn't they make it a habit themselves? If educators want students to make polite requests of each other instead of barking orders, shouldn't they practice the habit of making polite requests? Instead of hollering, "Stop that!" shouldn't we choose to say, "Please don't do that"? No teaching tool is more powerful than behaving in a way that supports what you do.

Summary

This book is meant to help make teaching and assessing in physical education easier and more efficient for both new and veteran physical educators. As you read the chapters that follow, keep in mind the information presented in this chapter—scoring with rubrics, threads in physical education, interactions, fitness routines, feedback, power of choice, music, and modeling. Begin thinking of ways in which you can incorporate the ideas and assessments presented here into units that you intend to develop or that you already have in place. Understanding and applying these ideas can help you use time more efficiently and help students get more out of each class period.

CHAPTER

Checkout: Daily Self-Assessment System

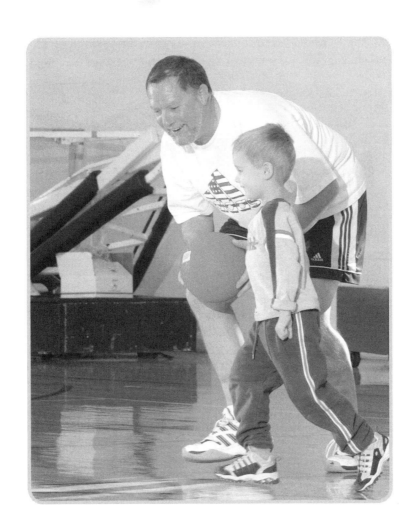

This chapter offers ideas about how to implement assessments that will give students a way to reflect on their daily performance based on clearly specified criteria. The chapter also includes ideas about how to incorporate knowledge assessments on the concept or skill focus of the unit. Using this system of assessment can quickly become a classroom routine that both you and your students will value. All the assessment forms discussed in this chapter are available for reproduction on the accompanying CD-ROM.

The Idea

Teaching kids the process of self-assessment and giving them opportunities to practice it help them to reflect on their daily performance and make positive changes. The checkout system provides students a structured way to reflect on their daily work in physical education, and you can use it at the end of every physical education class. In many instances, class ends and students rush off to their next class without having time to process what or how they did. One way to help students improve their class performance is to give them structured opportunities to reflect on it. The checkout system offers you a tool for student self-reflection that doesn't take a lot of time once established. This system helps students take responsibility for their learning, daily class performance, and, at times, behavior. It also gives you a place to start when having a conference with students and parents about performance. Does this system take time to set up at the beginning of each year? Definitely, but it's time well spent. If you have students for more than one year, less time is required in following years.

Many physical educators are concerned with the amount of contact time that they have with their students. The quality of the time spent is just as important as the quantity. Implementing a system such as this improves the quality of instructional time for both teachers and students. Students need only a few minutes to check out at the end of each class, and the process itself provides them with a way in which to reflect and focus on what is important for teaching and learning in physical education classes. Ultimately, the checkout system can help them make the connection between daily work habits and achievement.

Assessments

For students, checking out means that they rate themselves against predetermined criteria. The process is more powerful when students have helped to come up with the criteria. Three well-explained categories help keep the process manageable. Each class has a folder with a checkout sheet for each student. After each class period, students take their checkout sheets and shade in the number that corresponds with the skill listed. At the end of each trimester you and the student can clearly see in bar-graph form what skills he or she needs to focus on during the next trimester. You can combine some sort of point or grading system with this, but the real value is not in a grade written on a report card but in the process of learning self-assessment skills and taking steps in the direction of becoming a self-directed learner.

This chapter includes three kinds of checkout forms.

- One type of checkout sheet is designed to be used throughout an entire year.
- Another type is designed to be used for one unit of instruction.
- Cooperative groups or teams use the final checkout sheet to focus on the specific behaviors and skills necessary to work with others to achieve a common goal.

In addition, there are examples of content fill-ins that can be copied on the reverse side of the checkout sheets to incorporate content into the checkout process. The badminton unit in chapter 11 illustrates the process of using the checkout system for a unit.

Checkout Sheets

There are six daily checkout sheets available for use with your physical education classes. The following information describes each one. After reviewing them and looking at the forms at the end of the chapter, you will be able to choose the one that best suits your needs. For tips on using these forms, see "Putting It Into Practice: Checkout Sheets" on page 14.

- Physical Education Daily Checkout 1 (form 2.1) is an example of a checkout template that has been used with classes to give you an idea of a complete form. With guidance, students developed the categories and criteria, which you can use as printed.
- Physical Education Daily Checkout 2 (form 2.2) provides a blank template with the same categories, but the criteria for each category is blank so that you and your students can come up with the specifics as a team.
- Physical Education Daily Checkout 3 (form 2.3) is a checkout template that allows you and your students to determine what three categories and criteria are important for their classes. You can fill in a template after the group has come to consensus and photocopy the form for each student to use throughout the year.
- Physical Education Daily Checkout 4, 5, and 6 (forms 2.4 through 2.6) provide templates that you can use for daily checkout for just one unit of instruction. Again, three forms are supplied to allow the option of using the categories and criteria provided or creating your own criteria or categories.

Content Fill-Ins

After students understand the procedure, you can use the checkout system to target basic knowledge in content areas that are common to many units of instruction in physical education, such as health- and skill-related fitness concepts, social interactions, or application of concepts that govern movement. Using the checkout sheet for one unit allows the option of copying some content questions on the reverse side.

You can use Thinking About Flexibility (form 2.7), Thinking About Cardiorespiratory Fitness (form 2.8), Practicing Virtues (form 2.9), Thinking About Muscular Strength and Muscular Endurance (form 2.10), Thinking About Skill-Related Fitness (form 2.11), Thinking About Fitness Training (form 2.12), and Thinking About Physiological Changes (form 2.13) at the end of each class period to get students thinking about specific content information as well as their daily performance. At the bottom of each content fill-in is a formula to compute percent

accuracy. For tips on using these forms, see "Putting It Into Practice: Content Fill-Ins" on page 15.

Team Checkout

The versatility of the checkout system allows it to be used for cooperative groups or teams. How many times in physical education classes do kids work together in teams? For some children, learning how to work with others toward a common goal is a bigger challenge than mastering the physical skills to participate successfully. This is a wonderful time to take advantage of a group self-assessment system to help kids identify and work to improve the qualities that it takes to be productive in a team situation. Clearly spelled-out criteria used with a checkout sheet will help students become better at team skills because the target is defined and students are held accountable to work toward it. When students receive a chance to focus on clearly defined skills, they are more likely to hit their target. Physical Education Team Checkout (form 2.14) is a checkout template that you can use when students are working in cooperative groups or teams. For tips on using this form, see "Putting It Into Practice: Team Checkout" on page 15.

Setting Up Everyone for Success

Taking the time to teach students to self-assess against a predetermined set of criteria is key to successful implementation. Students spend a lot of time sitting and listening to class rules and procedures, especially at the beginning of the year. The following lessons provide a way to help students become familiar with the checkout system in an active way that will help them remember the categories and criteria. Using an activity like this will help set the tone of the class and help students learn what you will expect of them during every physical education class. The goal is to help them see the target more clearly so that they can hit it more often. Why not set up everyone to meet class expectations from the beginning? If you're going to hold students accountable for specific class habits and behaviors, you need to be sure that the students clearly understand what you expect of them.

On the pages that follow, you will find lists of ideas for putting each type of assessment form into practice with your students. The lists represent ways in which they have been used before and provide space for you to come up with other ways in which you might use them. Following the "Putting It Into Practice" sections, you will find lesson ideas that target some of the assessments in this chapter. The lessons can be used as written or modified to meet specific needs. The Class Expectations Lesson Sequence on page 16 lets students become familiar with the checkout system in an active way that will help them remember the categories and criteria. Using these lessons will help set the tone of the class and help students learn what you expect of them during every physical education class. The goal is to help them see the target more clearly so that they can hit it more often. Why not set up everyone to meet class expectations from the beginning? If you are going to hold students accountable for specific class habits and behaviors, you need to be sure that they clearly understand what you expect of them. Finally, you will find all of the forms referred to in this chapter. They are also found on the accompanying CD-ROM for easy printing and use.

Summary

Taking the extra time to help students become familiar with and practice daily habits that will help them experience success in physical education classes is well worth it. Getting students to think about and reflect on their daily performance is invaluable in the long run. When students understand what is expected, they become better students and your classes run more smoothly. Besides using the checkout system, you can use those few minutes at the end of the period to slip in some content review by using the reverse side of the checkout sheets.

PUTTING IT INTO PRACTICE

Checkout Sheets

▪ **Class folders**—All checkout sheets for one class are kept in a folder. At the end of the class period, instruct students to get their papers, shade in the appropriate numbers, and then get ready to leave class.

▪ **Reminders**—Sometimes the hardest category for students to grasp is "Doing quality work." Often they think that if they do not get everything right or do everything perfectly, they are not doing quality work. You can ease this confusion by taking a minute at the beginning of class to clarify just what doing quality work for the class period will look like. Do this according to the focus of the lesson. For instance, if students are working on dribbling skills, you could remind them that doing quality work during the lesson really means focusing on the skill cues for dribbling. Students may not always control the ball, but to do quality work, they simply need to focus on the skill cues that will help them improve.

▪ **Out the door**—When students hand in checkout sheets as they go out the door, you can glance at the sheets and talk with individual students if you have questions or concerns. If you need more time for a particular situation, schedule a one-on-one discussion.

▪ Other ways in which this type of assessment could be used:

_____

_____

_____

Content Fill-Ins

- **One at a time**—Instruct students to try to answer specific questions at the end of a class period, depending on the focus of the lesson.
- **All at the end**—All questions can be answered at the end of the unit.
- **Choices**—Allow students to choose the rate at which they will answer the questions given the allotted time and let them change those answers throughout the unit as they learn.
- **Pre- and postinstruction**—Have students attempt to answer all questions at the beginning of the unit and then check their answers against newly acquired knowledge.
- **Partners**—Students complete the questions with partners.
- Other ways in which this type of assessment could be used:

_____

_____

_____

Team Checkout

- **Consensus**—Distribute the team checkout sheets and call out the items on the list. Teams must come to consensus using the consensus decision-making process to make decisions about their scores.
- **Team facilitator**—Keep team checkout sheets for one class in a folder. At the end of the class period, instruct one team member to get the checkout sheet and facilitate making the decisions that the team needs to make.
- **Vote and discuss**—Each team member writes on a scrap of paper whether he or she thinks that the team deserves to shade in the box next to each of the items on the team checkout. After all team members have made a decision they put their votes in the center of the team. Team members discuss the results and decide on each item using the consensus decision-making process.
- Other ways in which this type of assessment could be used:

_____

_____

_____

Class Expectations Lesson Sequence

CONCEPT FOCUS

Quality work (QW), using time efficiently (TE), being a respectful and responsible class member (RR), practicing virtues (PV), expectations for class performance, virtues

SKILL FOCUS

Moving into open spaces, locomotor movements, variety of physical skills, checking out

EQUIPMENT AND MATERIALS

Upbeat music, CD player, a piece of scrap paper and a pencil for each student, flip chart or whiteboard, markers, music, eight Virtue Clue Cards (form 2.15), lined paper, equipment for stations in step 3, checkout sheets

TEACHING AND LEARNING ACTIVITIES

Step 1: Learning the Lingo

Setup
As students enter the gym ask them to find an open space.

Checkout Category Partners (20 to 25 Minutes)
Checkout Category Partners is an activity that will help students become familiar with the rules and procedures that you will hold them accountable for during physical education classes.

Directions

1. Tell students that they are going to play a memory game that will help them learn some of the rules and procedures for physical education class. Instruct them to move with control, using a locomotor movement of their choice, when the music starts. Point out the boundaries that will be used for classes and ask students to stay within those boundaries while they move. When the music stops they must stop wherever they are and listen for directions. During this activity you should review signals and formations that you use during class so that you can begin using time efficiently from the beginning.

2. Stop the music. When you have their attention ask them to take 10 giant steps in any direction and face another person who is close to them. As they face this person ask them to say the letters QW. Have some fun with it. Think of different ways for them to say QW. For instance, they could say QW in a high squeaky voice, say QW while giving a high five, and so forth. Make it fun and be enthusiastic. This type of activity has been used with young children, middle school students, and adult learners in workshops. Leading it with enthusiasm will engage the learners.

3. Tell students that they need to remember the person to whom they said QW because he or she is their QW partner. When the music starts again they will move into open spaces, but they must remember their QW partners. Ask them to be thinking about what the initials QW might stand for as they move. Play the music to signal students to move into open spaces. After a short time, stop the music and ask students to find their QW partners as fast as they can.

4. After they have done this and everyone is standing with his or her partner, ask them if they can come up with what QW stands for. Of course, you know that QW stands for quality work, and you could give them a hint of some sort to get them started. Tell them that partners who come to consensus on what QW stands for can sit down. After a few minutes call on students

who are sitting to share what they think QW might mean. If they are having difficulty, lead them with questions and hints to come up with the correct answer.

5. Follow the same procedure for the letters TE (using time efficiently), RR (being a respectful and responsible class member), and PV (practicing virtues). Between each set of letters play a little memory and movement game by calling out the initials in random order and seeing if students can find their partners. At the end, call them quickly in succession and see how fast students can find their respective partners. You will need to stand in for any student who is absent so that he or she will be able to catch up during the next class period.

Note: For this activity, letters correspond with the categories in the checkout template shown in Physical Education Daily Checkout 1 (form 2.1). If you choose different categories, you will need to make corresponding changes in the letters.

Closure (10 to 12 Minutes)

Gather students into a circle and ask them if they can think of four things that they should remember when participating in physical education classes this year (doing quality work, using time efficiently, being a respectful and responsible class member, and practicing virtues). They should quickly be able to come up with the four that you are looking for. Instruct them that on the signal to go, they should give each of their partners a high five and say, "Great work today." On a small piece of scrap paper, they should record the names of their partners for each set of letters, put their own name on the back, and hand them to you on the way out of class.

Step 2: Remembering and Reviewing

Setup

Set up the flip chart or whiteboard outside the movement area. You will also need a box of pencils.

Partner Review (10 to 15 Minutes)

This activity will help students recall the previous lesson.

Directions

1. As students walk into class, have them find an open space. Ask them to turn and without moving from their spot reach or stretch as far as they can in the direction of their QW partner. Ask if anyone remembers what QW stands for. Follow this procedure for TE, RR, and PV. They can consult their list of partners from the last class if they forget.

2. Instruct them that when the music starts, you will begin calling partners and that they need to find that partner as fast as they can, give a high five, and then listen for the next set of letters. Mix up the order to get them thinking.

Class Focus Tag (10 Minutes)

This activity combines the checkout categories with a fun game activity that will further cement the categories in students' minds.

Directions

1. Begin with all students in open spaces. On the signal to begin, students attempt to tag as many people as possible with one major rule: They cannot tag their QW, TE, RR, or PV partners.

2. If tagged, students stand in the high-five position (standing up with one hand in the air ready for a high five).

3. To be set free and able to resume tagging, students must receive a high five from one of their partners (QW, TE, RR, or PV). This is a fun way to use the partners. This game will be used again for movement breaks during the next part of the lesson.

Coming Up With Criteria (10 to 15 Minutes)

You should involve students in setting the criteria for each of the checkout categories. This activity will guide them through the process.

Directions

1. Ask students to circle up around the flip chart or whiteboard sitting next to their QW partners. Acting as a facilitator, lead the class in coming up with the definitions of the categories identified as being a focus for daily work.

2. On the first sheet of paper write the heading "Doing quality work." With their QW partners, students have a minute or two to come up with what they think doing quality work means in terms of their work in physical education class. Ask them to use positive language. For instance, they might say, "No interrupting," but a positive alternative would be to say, "Be a respectful listener." If they don't understand, ask if anyone could come up with an example to share with the class. Record what they come up with on the board. Use this opportunity to talk about the importance of practicing respect while working with a partner.

3. Follow the same procedure with the RR and TE partnerships, giving students a break after each period of brainstorming with a quick one-minute round of the tag game you just played. This creates an opportunity to point out how well students can transition from activity to a circle.

Closure (1 to 2 Minutes)

Gather students together and ask them if anyone knows what a virtue is (personal, positive qualities that people can develop to become a good person). Facilitate the group until everyone understands a definition. Ask them to be thinking between now and the next meeting about which virtues or values are important to practice during physical education class.

Step 3: Practicing Virtues

Setup

Create the stations around the room. The stations can be of any type because the focus of the lesson is on the virtues that students will be practicing throughout the year to help everyone have a positive, productive learning experience in physical education. The best approach is to organize a few stations where students practice individual skills, a few that involve a little competition, and a few that require cooperation. Place one of the Virtue Clue Cards (form 2.15) and a pencil at eight of the stations. Each partnership will need a lined piece of paper that they carry with them to record their answers.

Clue Card Stations (30 to 40 Minutes)

By participating in these stations and guessing what each of the virtues are, students will start to build the vocabulary that you would like them to use in class.

Directions

1. As students enter the room have them sit in a designated area with their PV (practicing virtues) partners.

2. Quickly give instructions for the activities at each station.

3. Tell students that they will find a Virtue Clue Card at eight of the stations. The card will provide the first letter of a virtue, lines representing the number of letters in the virtue, and a clue to help them figure out what it is.

4. Students will move to a station, read the clue card if it is one of the eight stations with clue cards, perform the activity, and stop on the signal. If the station does not have a clue card, students just perform the activity.

5. On the signal to stop activity, partners need to come to consensus on what the virtue for that station might be and record it on their paper. They then rotate to the next station.

   This is a good opportunity to have students review or learn how to use the consensus decision-making process that you would like them to use. See the example on page 7 in chapter 1. Making decisions with others is a skill that students need to practice. If a procedure is in place for students to use whenever they must make a decision and you hold them accountable for using it, classes will run more smoothly.

6. After each group has visited all stations, have each partnership bring the clue card from their last station to one area. Students can take turns reading the clues and volunteering answers. Facilitate the group in coming up with the complete list. Record each answer on the board or flip chart. The answers to the clue cards appear in the appendix.

Closure (1 to 2 Minutes)

Ask students to think about the stations where they last worked. Then ask them to identify a virtue that they could practice to help both partners experience success and improve skills in the different situations. Making connections between the virtues to practice and cooperative, competitive, partner, and individual physical activities is the first step for students to make in developing those qualities. Virtues or values are the threads that bind everything together for smooth, peaceful classes. Using this type of lesson to set up the process at the beginning of the year will lead to classes that are more productive. This lesson also helps build vocabulary.

Step 4: Putting Everything Together

Setup

Have checkout sheets and pencils alongside the activity area. As students enter the gym, have them get a paper, put their name on it, sit in a circle, and look it over until everyone is settled.

Review (10 to 15 Minutes)

Quickly review the previous lessons before beginning the first lesson of the unit that you will be teaching to prepare students to use the checkout system at the end of every class period.

Directions

1. Explain that after each class period, they will be using their checkout sheets to self-assess whether they met the criteria for doing quality work as defined by the criteria. To start, have students sit next to their QW (quality work) partners and ask them to take turns reading the criteria listed under doing quality work. Tell them that if at the end of class they decide that they met the criteria for doing quality work, they will shade in the number 1. Demonstrate this on a blank checkout template for everyone to see.

2. Follow the same procedures for TE (using time efficiently) and RR (being a respectful and responsible class member) partners.

3. After finishing all three categories, explain that practicing the virtues that they learned about during the last class period will help everyone in class meet the criteria for each class period.

4. When you feel that students have a clear understanding of how the checkout sheets work, start the first lesson of the unit that you plan to teach.

5. Have students use the sheet at the end of class. Check to be sure that all students understand as they hand in the sheets on their way out the door. After a few class periods, this system will move quickly and become an established routine. You may at times want to revisit the criteria to bring attention to specific categories and criteria.

Physical Education Daily Checkout 1

Name _____

TRIMESTER 1

1	2	3
1	2	3
1	2	3
1	2	3
1	2	3
1	2	3
1	2	3
1	2	3
1	2	3
1	2	3
1	2	3
1	2	3
1	2	3
1	2	3
1	2	3
1	2	3
1	2	3
1	2	3
1	2	3
1	2	3
1	2	3
1	2	3
1	2	3
1	2	3
1	2	3
1	2	3

TRIMESTER 2

1	2	3
1	2	3
1	2	3
1	2	3
1	2	3
1	2	3
1	2	3
1	2	3
1	2	3
1	2	3
1	2	3
1	2	3
1	2	3
1	2	3
1	2	3
1	2	3
1	2	3
1	2	3
1	2	3
1	2	3
1	2	3
1	2	3
1	2	3
1	2	3
1	2	3
1	2	3

TRIMESTER 3

1	2	3
1	2	3
1	2	3
1	2	3
1	2	3
1	2	3
1	2	3
1	2	3
1	2	3
1	2	3
1	2	3
1	2	3
1	2	3
1	2	3
1	2	3
1	2	3
1	2	3
1	2	3
1	2	3
1	2	3
1	2	3
1	2	3
1	2	3
1	2	3
1	2	3
1	2	3

(continued)

Directions: Shade in the number that represents each skill if you feel that you met the standard for performance. Be sure that you are practicing honesty when you shade in each number. You may be asked to explain your choices.

1. Doing quality work

    • I remained on task and focused on the specific skill cues for today's skill or lesson.

    • I worked to improve skills today.

    • I persevered by having an "I can" attitude.

2. Being a respectful and responsible classmate

    • I listened to my classmates and made eye contact. I didn't interrupt.

    • I tried to be creative and open-minded.

    • I gave effort, energy, and enthusiasm to the tasks.

    • When a decision needed to be made, I didn't give orders. I used the consensus decision-making process.

    • If involved in a conflict, I used conflict resolution skills, "I" statements, and a calm, soft voice instead of a loud, angry voice.

3. Using time efficiently

    • I carried out directions and transitions quickly and quietly.

    • I responded to signals immediately and appropriately.

From *Physical Education Assessment Toolkit* by Liz Giles-Brown, 2006, Champaign, IL: Human Kinetics.

Physical Education Daily Checkout 2

Name _____

TRIMESTER 1

1	2	3
1	2	3
1	2	3
1	2	3
1	2	3
1	2	3
1	2	3
1	2	3
1	2	3
1	2	3
1	2	3
1	2	3
1	2	3
1	2	3
1	2	3
1	2	3
1	2	3
1	2	3
1	2	3
1	2	3
1	2	3
1	2	3
1	2	3

TRIMESTER 2

1	2	3
1	2	3
1	2	3
1	2	3
1	2	3
1	2	3
1	2	3
1	2	3
1	2	3
1	2	3
1	2	3
1	2	3
1	2	3
1	2	3
1	2	3
1	2	3
1	2	3
1	2	3
1	2	3
1	2	3
1	2	3
1	2	3
1	2	3

TRIMESTER 3

1	2	3
1	2	3
1	2	3
1	2	3
1	2	3
1	2	3
1	2	3
1	2	3
1	2	3
1	2	3
1	2	3
1	2	3
1	2	3
1	2	3
1	2	3
1	2	3
1	2	3
1	2	3
1	2	3
1	2	3
1	2	3
1	2	3
1	2	3

(continued)

Directions: Shade in the number that represents each skill if you feel that you met the standard for performance. Be sure that you are practicing honesty when you shade in each number. You may be asked to explain your choices.

1. Doing quality work

- _____
  _____
  _____
- _____
  _____
  _____
- _____
  _____
  _____

2. Being a respectful and responsible classmate

- _____
  _____
  _____
- _____
  _____
  _____
- _____
  _____

3. Using time efficiently

- _____
  _____
  _____
- _____
  _____
  _____
- _____
  _____

Physical Education Daily Checkout 3

Name _____

TRIMESTER 1

I	2	3
I	2	3
I	2	3
I	2	3
I	2	3
I	2	3
I	2	3
I	2	3
I	2	3
I	2	3
I	2	3
I	2	3
I	2	3
I	2	3
I	2	3
I	2	3
I	2	3
I	2	3
I	2	3
I	2	3
I	2	3
I	2	3
I	2	3
I	2	3

TRIMESTER 2

I	2	3
I	2	3
I	2	3
I	2	3
I	2	3
I	2	3
I	2	3
I	2	3
I	2	3
I	2	3
I	2	3
I	2	3
I	2	3
I	2	3
I	2	3
I	2	3
I	2	3
I	2	3
I	2	3
I	2	3
I	2	3
I	2	3
I	2	3
I	2	3

TRIMESTER 3

I	2	3
I	2	3
I	2	3
I	2	3
I	2	3
I	2	3
I	2	3
I	2	3
I	2	3
I	2	3
I	2	3
I	2	3
I	2	3
I	2	3
I	2	3
I	2	3
I	2	3
I	2	3
I	2	3
I	2	3
I	2	3
I	2	3
I	2	3
I	2	3

(continued)

Directions: Shade in the number that represents each skill if you feel that you met the standard for performance. Be sure that you are practicing honesty when you shade in each number. You may be asked to explain your choices.

1. _____

   • _____
   _____
   _____

   • _____
   _____
   _____

   • _____
   _____
   _____

2. _____

   • _____
   _____
   _____

   • _____
   _____
   _____

   • _____
   _____
   _____

3. _____

   • _____
   _____
   _____

   • _____
   _____
   _____

   • _____
   _____
   _____

From *Physical Education Assessment Toolkit* by Liz Giles-Brown, 2006, Champaign, IL: Human Kinetics.

Physical Education Daily Checkout 4

Name _____ **Unit** _____

Directions: Shade in the number that represents each skill if you feel that you met the standard for performance. Be sure that you are practicing honesty when you shade in each number. You may be asked to explain your choices.

I	2	3
I	2	3
I	2	3
I	2	3
I	2	3
I	2	3
I	2	3
I	2	3
I	2	3
I	2	3
I	2	3
I	2	3
I	2	3
I	2	3
I	2	3
I	2	3
I	2	3
I	2	3
I	2	3
I	2	3
I	2	3
I	2	3
I	2	3
I	2	3
I	2	3

1. Doing quality work

- I remained on task and focused on the specific skill cues for today's skill or lesson.
- I worked to improve skills today.
- I persevered by having an "I can" attitude.

2. Being a respectful and responsible classmate

- I listened to my classmates and made eye contact. I didn't interrupt.
- I tried to be creative and open-minded.
- I gave effort, energy, and enthusiasm to the tasks.
- When a decision needed to be made, I didn't give orders. I used the consensus decision-making process.
- If involved in a conflict, I used conflict resolution skills, "I" statements, and a calm, soft voice instead of a loud, angry voice.

3. Using time efficiently

- I carried out directions and transitions quickly and quietly.
- I responded to signals immediately and appropriately.

Physical Education Daily Checkout 5

Name _____ **Unit** _____

Directions: Shade in the number that represents each skill if you feel that you met the standard for performance. Be sure that you are practicing honesty when you shade in each number. You may be asked to explain your choices.

1	2	3
1	2	3
1	2	3
1	2	3
1	2	3
1	2	3
1	2	3
1	2	3
1	2	3
1	2	3
1	2	3
1	2	3
1	2	3
1	2	3
1	2	3
1	2	3
1	2	3
1	2	3
1	2	3
1	2	3
1	2	3
1	2	3
1	2	3
1	2	3
1	2	3
1	2	3

1. Doing quality work

- _____
- _____
- _____

2. Being a respectful and responsible classmate

- _____
- _____
- _____

3. Using time efficiently

- _____
- _____
- _____

Physical Education Daily Checkout 6

Name _____ **Unit** _____

Directions: Shade in the number that represents each skill if you feel that you met the standard for performance. Be sure that you are practicing honesty when you shade in each number. You may be asked to explain your choices.

I	2	3
I	2	3
I	2	3
I	2	3
I	2	3
I	2	3
I	2	3
I	2	3
I	2	3
I	2	3
I	2	3
I	2	3
I	2	3
I	2	3
I	2	3
I	2	3
I	2	3
I	2	3
I	2	3
I	2	3
I	2	3
I	2	3
I	2	3
I	2	3

I. _____

_____

• _____

_____

• _____

_____

• _____

_____

2. _____

_____

• _____

_____

• _____

_____

• _____

_____

3. _____

_____

• _____

_____

• _____

_____

• _____

_____

Thinking About Flexibility

Name _____

Directions: Complete the following statements about flexibility by using the words provided.

1. Flexibility is being able to use your muscles to bend, _____, and twist as far as possible.

2. When you stretch, your muscles might feel tight but they should not _____.
Always stretch as far as you can without feeling _____.

3. When you do static flexibility exercises, stretch slowly without _____.

4. Always do _____ exercises for all the muscles that you will use in an activity.

5. Flexibility exercises keep muscles _____ and flexible instead of short and _____.

6. People who are very flexible are able to use their_____ fully.

7. People with healthful levels of flexibility have fewer sore or _____ muscles.

8. _____ muscles will not stretch as far as warm muscles. Warming up with light activity before stretching is a good idea.

stretch	hurt	bouncing	long	tight
joints	injured	cold	pain	flexibility

Scoring: The number of correct answers _____ divided by the number of possible answers _____ equals the percentage of correct answers _____.

Thinking About Cardiorespiratory Fitness

Name _____

Directions: Complete the following statements about cardiorespiratory fitness by using the words provided.

1. People with healthful levels of cardiorespiratory fitness are able to be active for a long _____ .

2. Cardiorespiratory fitness requires a strong _____, healthy lungs, and clear blood vessels.

3. Before participating in cardiorespiratory fitness activities, you should warm up to bring about a _____ increase in breathing and heart rate.

4. When participating in cardiorespiratory activities, your body uses _____ and fats for energy.

5. During cardiorespiratory activities your circulatory system and _____ system work together to deliver food and _____ to your working muscles.

6. Choosing to participate regularly in cardiorespiratory fitness activities when you are young and throughout your life may help reduce the risk of heart disease and other illnesses when you are _____ .

7. Cardiorespiratory activities give your heart and _____ a workout to help them stay healthy.

8. _____, swimming, power walking, and playing tag are all examples of cardiorespiratory activities.

9. Choosing cardiorespiratory activities that you enjoy and participating in them at least _____ times each week is a gift that you give your heart, lungs, and blood vessels.

time	heart	gradual	jogging	respiratory
oxygen	older	lungs	three	carbohydrates

Scoring: The number of correct answers _____ divided by the number of possible answers _____ equals the percentage of correct answers _____ .

Practicing Virtues

Name _____

Directions: As we work to improve skills and fitness during this unit, we will also be working on some virtues essential to success in physical education. After each virtue, list one thing that you did or said or saw someone else do or say that shows evidence of this virtue. You do not have to complete the list in any specific order.

DATE

__/__/__ I practiced respect when I _____

_____

__/__/__ I practiced responsibility when I _____

_____

__/__/__ I practiced perseverance when I _____

_____

__/__/__ I practiced self-discipline when I _____

_____

__/__/__ I practiced honesty when I _____

_____

__/__/__ I practiced compassion when I _____

_____

__/__/__ I practiced courage when I _____

_____

__/__/__ I practiced trustworthiness when I _____

_____

Scoring: The number of complete answers _____ divided by the number of possible answers _____ equals the percentage of complete answers _____.

From *Physical Education Assessment Toolkit* by Liz Giles-Brown, 2006, Champaign, IL: Human Kinetics.

Thinking About Muscular Strength and Muscular Endurance

Name _____

Directions: Complete the following statements about muscular strength and endurance by using the words provided.

1. Strength is being able to produce a lot of _____ with one strong movement.

2. Endurance is the ability to use the muscles over and over without getting _____.

3. People with healthful levels of muscular strength and endurance have better _____.

4. Muscular strength and endurance are both components of _____- related fitness.

5. When you use your abdominal muscles to perform many curl-ups, you are performing a muscular _____ activity.

6. When you try to throw a ball as far as you can, you are using muscular _____.

7. Muscular strength is a _____ of energy. It involves using the muscles one time in a forceful movement.

8. Riding a bicycle a long distance requires a lot of muscular endurance in your _____.

9. Hitting a ball with a bat a long distance requires strength in the muscles of your _____ body.

10. To build muscular strength and endurance, you can choose exercises that require your muscles to do _____ than they normally do.

tired	force	posture	health	endurance
strength	burst	legs	upper	more

Scoring: The number of correct answers _____ divided by the number of possible answers _____ equals the percentage of correct answers _____.

From *Physical Education Assessment Toolkit* by Liz Giles-Brown, 2006, Champaign, IL: Human Kinetics.

Thinking About Skill-Related Fitness

Name _____

Directions: Complete the following statements about skill-related fitness by using the words provided.

1. A _____ movement is smooth and efficient with little wasted motion.

2. When someone is able to change direction quickly when moving at top speed we say that he or she has a lot of _____.

3. Moving from one place to another in the shortest time possible requires great _____.

4. In a powerful movement a person uses strong _____ in one explosive act.

5. _____ balance requires a person to maintain equilibrium while still.

6. Dynamic _____ involves maintaining equilibrium while moving.

7. The _____ is a movement that requires power.

8. When playing defense against someone who is able to change _____ quickly, you must be agile.

9. A juggler must have high levels of _____ to keep all those balls in the air.

10. Many physical activities involve different combinations of health-related fitness components as well as _____-related fitness components.

coordinated	speed	static	direction	agility
force	balance	skill	coordination	standing broad jump

Scoring: The number of correct answers _____ divided by the number of possible answers _____ equals the percentage of correct answers _____.

From *Physical Education Assessment Toolkit* by Liz Giles-Brown, 2006, Champaign, IL: Human Kinetics.

Thinking About Fitness Training

Name _____

Directions: Complete the following statements about fitness training by using the words provided.

1. Duration refers to how _____ you work.

2. Frequency refers to how _____ you work.

3. Intensity refers to how _____ you work.

4. Overload refers to doing _____ than you are used to doing.

5. Progression refers to _____ the amount of work gradually.

6. The intensity of a cardiorespiratory workout is measured by your _____.

7. If you would like to build muscular strength and endurance, you must _____ the muscles by making them work harder.

8. To maintain good cardiorespiratory fitness, you should plan to exercise at least three times each week for at least 20 minutes at moderate _____.

9. During the first week of a new fitness plan, Jeff did 20 curl-ups every other day and found that he could do it fairly easily. He should overload his muscles by doing 22 to 25 curl-ups the following week if he wants to improve _____.

10. To determine the best intensity of your cardiorespiratory workout, you will need to calculate your _____.

long	hard	often	heart rate	more
overload	intensity	increasing	muscular endurance	target heart rate

Scoring: The number of correct answers _____ divided by the number of possible answers _____ equals the percentage of correct answers _____.

From *Physical Education Assessment Toolkit* by Liz Giles-Brown, 2006, Champaign, IL: Human Kinetics.

Thinking About Physiological Changes

Name _____

Directions: During cardiorespiratory activity, physiological changes occur in the body. Circle T for true or F for false according to whether each change happens during exercise.

1. T F   Heart rate decreases.

2. T F   The heart pumps more blood with each beat.

3. T F   Blood flow to the working muscles increases.

4. T F   Blood flow to the lungs decreases.

5. T F   Breathing rate increases.

6. T F   Blood flow to the heart muscle itself increases.

7. T F   Blood flow to the digestive organs decreases.

8. T F   Blood flow to the skin increases to carry away excess heat and cool the body.

9. T F   The body uses carbohydrates and fat for energy at a slower rate.

10. T F   Blood carries oxygen and food to working muscles at a faster rate.

Scoring: The number of correct answers _____ divided by the number of possible answers _____ equals the percentage of correct answers _____.

Physical Education Team Checkout

Name _____ **Unit** _____

Directions: Shade in the number that represents each skill if you feel that your team met the standard for performance. Be sure that you are practicing honesty when you shade in each number. You may be asked to explain your choices.

1	2	3
1	2	3
1	2	3
1	2	3
1	2	3
1	2	3
1	2	3
1	2	3
1	2	3
1	2	3
1	2	3
1	2	3
1	2	3
1	2	3
1	2	3
1	2	3
1	2	3
1	2	3
1	2	3
1	2	3
1	2	3
1	2	3
1	2	3
1	2	3
1	2	3

1. _____
   _____
   • _____
   _____
   • _____
   _____
   • _____
   _____

2. _____
   _____
   • _____
   _____
   • _____
   _____
   • _____
   _____

3. _____
   _____
   • _____
   _____
   • _____
   _____
   • _____
   _____

Virtue Clue Cards

You practice this virtue when dealing with all people. Sometimes it's hard when you are having a disagreement, but someone who practices this virtue will treat all people with consideration.

R _ _ _ _ _ _

People who practice this virtue are willing to accept the consequences for their own actions whether those consequences are bad or good.

R _ _ _ _ _ _ _ _ _ _ _ _ _

This virtue is a voice inside your head that says, "If at first you don't succeed, try, try again." This virtue doesn't let you give up.

P _ _ _ _ _ _ _ _ _ _ _

You use this virtue to manage your behavior and help you control yourself. This virtue is the one that tells you to do your homework before you go outside to play.

S _ _ _ - d _ _ _ _ _ _ _ _ _

If you regularly practice this virtue, you are always truthful no matter what, even if it means that you might get into trouble.

H _ _ _ _ _ _

When you practice this virtue, you try to understand how another person feels in certain situations. This ability helps you care for others.

C _ _ _ _ _ _ _ _ _

When you are afraid, you will call on this virtue to do what you know you should do or need to do.

C _ _ _ _ _ _

People who possess this virtue are dependable. You can always trust that they will do the right thing.

T _ _ _ _ _ _ _ _ _ _ _ _ _ _

3

CHAPTER

Setting Goals and Reflecting on Performance

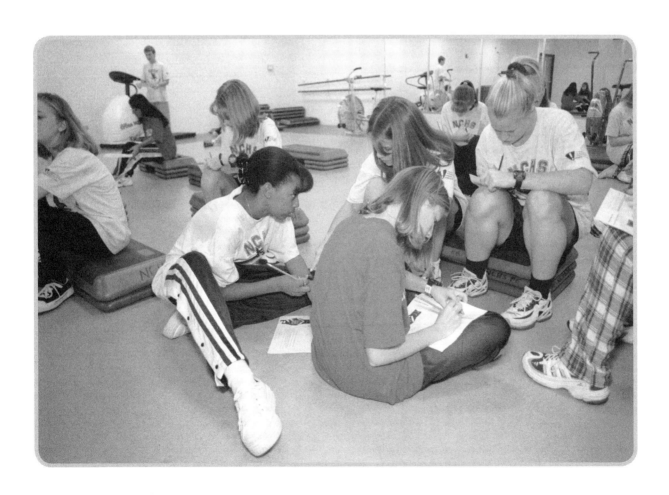

This chapter deals with the idea of having students set personal goals and reflect on their performance in physical education class. Several different types of assessment templates are provided to help you teach your students the important task of setting personal goals and learning how to reflect on performance in an objective way. As with most of the assessments in this book, you can use them with any unit of instruction. All assessment forms discussed in this chapter are available for reproduction on the accompanying CD-ROM.

The Idea

The first part of this chapter deals with personal goal setting. Some children and adults are natural goal setters, but not everyone is born with that ability. Some people need to be guided through a process. Physical education class is an excellent place for children to practice the process of setting goals. The practice of personal goal setting helps make the learning process more personal and therefore more meaningful for students. When students can make clear connections between what they are learning in class and their own lives, they will be more able to focus on the target. We all have many goals and objectives for our students. By taking the time to guide them through the goal-setting process, we can discover what is important to them.

The second part of this chapter is dedicated to having students reflect on different areas of their learning. When we ask students to reflect honestly on what they have learned or how they have performed, we are holding them accountable. The use of guided reflections in physical education is a powerful tool. Reflection gets kids thinking about their learning in physical education and helps them appreciate their successes as well as what they might need to do to improve. The daily assessment templates in chapter 2 serve as a way for students to reflect on their daily performance. The assessment templates provided in this chapter can be used to target specific skills learned and practiced in physical education classes.

Assessments

Two types of assessments are provided. Unit objectives will determine which one to use.

- Goal-setting and reflection assessments require students to set goals at the beginning of the unit, revisit the goals throughout the unit, and then reflect on their performance in relationship to their personal goals at the end of the unit.

- Guided reflection assessments provide you with different ways in which you can guide students to reflect on different aspects of the unit that they just participated in. They do not include a goal-setting portion.

Setting Goals and Reflecting

Setting Goals for Improvement (form 3.1), Working to Improve Our Community (form 3.2), and Setting Goals and Reflecting (form 3.3) are all assessments that involve students in setting personal goals and then reflecting on those goals at the end of the unit. This type of assessment is easy to use with a wide variety of ages. The depth of students' responses will depend on their age to some degree. The second portion of this type of assessment is set up to help students reflect on their personal goals and other areas of their performance during the unit.

The rubrics that accompany each of the assessments in this section are the same. They focus on the specificity and completeness of each response. All teachers struggle with students in this area. With some communication, teachers in other subject areas could focus on this area as well. When teachers begin thinking about education as a whole instead of seeing only their part, students will benefit. For tips on using these forms, see "Putting It Into Practice: Setting Goals and Reflecting" on page 41.

Guided Reflection

Unit Reflections 1 (form 3.4), Unit Reflections 2 (form 3.5), Reflecting on My Work in Physical Education (form 3.6), and Reflections Quick Check (form 3.7) involve reflecting on work done during the unit without including the goal-setting portion of the assessment. They provide a variety of ways in which students can think about their work during the unit. Although these assessments are given at the end of the unit, students should have a chance to review what it is they will be reflecting on near the beginning. This practice will sharpen their focus as they work. It's all part of beginning with the end.

Setting Up Everyone for Success

Students must know several things to be successful goal setters and reflectors. The most important of these is the vocabulary. If students aren't familiar with the terms and how they are being used, they will not be successful with these types of assessments. They must first know the difference between a realistic goal and an unrealistic goal. Although learning to set clear, realistic goals takes time, developing the skill is definitely worth it. Students also need to know the difference between a specific, measurable goal and one that is vague or general. Using some of the lesson activities listed in this section will help students become familiar with the vocabulary so that they can successfully complete the assessments.

On the pages that follow, you will find a list of ideas for putting each type of assessment form into practice with your students. The list represents ways in which they have been used before and provides space for you to come up with other ways in which you might use them. Following the "Putting It Into Practice" section, you will find lesson ideas that target some of the assessments in this chapter. The lessons can be used as written or modified to meet specific needs. The Setting Goals and Reflecting Lesson Sequence on page 43 offers ideas about how you might incorporate this type of assessment into any unit you are teaching. After students have gone through this process once, the next time this type of assessment is used it will take less instructional time to implement. Finally, you will find all of the forms referred to in this chapter. They are also found on the accompanying CD-ROM for easy printing and use.

Summary

Taking time to deal with personal goal setting and reflections is time well spent. Helping students develop this life skill will help them focus their work not only in physical education but also in other areas of their lives. They will learn to set meaningful, specific, realistic goals and be able to reflect on what has happened so that they can make changes for the future.

PUTTING IT INTO PRACTICE

Setting Goals and Reflecting

- **Goal setting on the way**—When students move from their classroom to the gym for physical education class, you can start the goal-setting process by giving students the task of setting a personal goal for the class period. For each unit the theme for the daily goal could be different. For the first month of school, students could set specific personal goals based on using class time efficiently. In other units, personal goals might be related to the skills that the students are working on. As students make their way into the gym, you can instruct them to share their goal with one other person, and on the way out they could visit again with their chosen classmate and tell whether they met their goal for the day. Alternatively, students could quickly tell you their goal on the way in and then report to you whether they met it on the way out.

- **Practicing reflections**—Getting students to understand what reflecting means can be built into a class ritual before you use the reflection assessment. As students head back to class from the gym, you can prompt them to reflect on a specific part of class. When they arrive in the classroom take a few minutes to let students volunteer their responses. Alternatively,

(continued)

you could give processing partners a chance to share their reflections for one or two minutes. This method doesn't take much time, and it can serve as an effective transition back into the classroom. Some classroom teachers might even incorporate it into a writing exercise that focuses on something that they are working on in the classroom (writing complete sentences, using punctuation correctly, using descriptive language, using parts of speech, and so on).

- **Placement**—If you choose one of these assessment templates for a unit, you must decide where to introduce it. You should have at least one lesson before having students set their goals so that they have a working understanding of what the unit will entail. If students are unclear, their goals will have less meaning.

- **Be specific**—Taking time to go over how to set a specific, measurable goal is well worth the effort. Students need to learn how to set specific goals. This process may take a bit of time, but goal setting is a skill that students will be able to use throughout their lives.

- **Review reflections**—After students set their personal goals, review the reflection portion of the assessment so that students know what will be expected at the end of the unit. This activity primes students and directs their thoughts toward the target.

- **Share**—After setting their goals, students can take a minute to share with a partner their personal goal and why they set it.

- **Revisit**—Be sure to have students revisit their goals throughout the unit so that they don't forget them. One way to do this is to have students look at their goals and share with a partner how they are progressing or why they set that particular goal.

- **Homework**—At the end of the unit, students can take the assessment sheet home and complete it as a homework assignment.

- **Stations**—You can set up stations around the gym and have one be the completion of the goal-setting and reflection sheet. When students are at that station, students complete their assessment.

- Other ways that this type of assessment could be used:

_____

_____

_____

Setting Goals and Reflecting Lesson Sequence

CONCEPT FOCUS

Specific versus general, movement concepts related to unit being taught

SKILL FOCUS

Setting specific goals, physical skills related to unit being taught

EQUIPMENT AND MATERIALS

One Setting Goals and Reflecting sheet (form 3.3) per student (with the information for numbers 1 and 2 filled in before copying it for student use), other equipment related to unit being taught

TEACHING AND LEARNING ACTIVITIES

Step 1: Becoming Familiar With the Form

During this step in the process, students will become familiar with the assessment form used for goal setting and reflecting.

Directions

1. As students enter the gym give each one a copy of Setting Goals and Reflecting (form 3.3). Ask them to take the paper and walk around the perimeter of the room.

2. Each time they reach a corner of the room, they stop moving forward, step in place, and read one part of the paper. For instance, at the first corner they will read number 1, at the second corner they will read number 2, and so on.

3. If they finish reading and you have not yet stopped the activity, tell them to perform one of their fitness routines (flexibility or muscular endurance) until you signal them to stop. Chapter 2 contains in-depth information about establishing fitness routines.

Step 2: Introducing Goal Setting

During this step in the process, students will begin to develop an understanding of goal setting in physical education.

Directions

1. Go over numbers 1 and 2 on Setting Goals and Reflecting (form 3.3), with students following along. Tell students that you have designed lessons that will help them reach the goals that you have set for everyone but that they should also set personal goals.

2. Quickly pair up students by having them turn to someone directly beside them and ask that person to come up with two reasons why it might be important to set personal goals.

3. After a few minutes ask students to share what they came up with.

4. Tell students that at the end of the class period after you have introduced the skills that they will be working on, they will complete number 3 on their sheets. They will need to be able to set a specific, realistic personal goal and tell why they chose that goal for themselves.

5. Tell students that you are going to state two goals and that you will be asking them whether the goals are specific or not: (a) I want to get better at golf; (b) I want to improve my golf swing so that I can hit the ball within 2 feet (60 centimeters) of my target three times out of five. Take volunteers to answer. Talk for a moment about specific versus general goals.

6. Have students place their papers out of the way and proceed with the activities that you have planned for the unit.

Note: This step may take a while the first time you use a goal-setting and reflecting assessment, but after that everything will go much more quickly.

Step 3: Setting the Goals

During this step in the process, students will set their personal goals.

Directions

1. At the close of class ask students to get the goal-setting sheet that you introduced at the beginning of the class.
2. Direct their attention to number 3. Have them move to an open space to set a personal goal and write it down. They also must state a specific reason why they chose that particular goal.
3. Read the reflection portion of the assessment sheet with them and go over the rubric so that they understand how they will be scored.
4. Let them know that you will look over their goals before the next class period to be sure that their goals are specific and realistic.

Step 4: Revisiting

During this step in the process, students revisit their goals and think about what they will need to do to reach them.

Directions

1. At appropriate times during the unit you need to let students revisit their goals so that they remember what they decided on. This activity takes only a minute and can be done during a warm-up or closure.
2. Do not let students change their goals at this time. The goal-setting process should be a learning experience. Setting unrealistic goals is OK. Students will learn from their mistakes and set goals that are more realistic next time.

Step 5: Reflecting

During this step in the process, students revisit their goals for the last time and reflect on them as well as on the other items on the assessment.

Directions

1. At the end of the unit hand out the goal setting and reflecting sheets and go over the reflection portion of the assessment.
2. Students can finish this portion either during class or as a homework assignment.
3. Be sure that students understand the rubric and the importance of being specific with their answers.
4. Correct the papers outside of class and return them to students during the following class period. If anyone has a specific question about his or her work, set up a time to talk about it one on one.

Setting Goals for Improvement

Name _____ **Date** _____

BEFORE YOU START

1. We are beginning a _____ unit. We will be working to improve the following skills:

_____

_____

Please take a few minutes and think about what your strengths and weaknesses might be in this area.

2. I feel that I am very good at _____

_____

_____

3. I feel that I need more practice on _____

_____

_____

Now take some time to set a specific, measurable, realistic goal.

4. By the end of this unit I would like to be able to _____

_____

_____

AFTER YOU FINISH

5. Did you reach the goal that you set? _____

_____

_____

6. How do you know? Be specific with your evidence. _____

_____

_____

Assessment: Your work will be scored according to the criteria in the following rubric. Use this information to self-assess your work before you hand it in.

4	Excellent work! You went above and beyond!	Answers are specific and complete. Artwork, specific examples, or details that support answers are included.
3	Good work. Everything is here!	Answers are specific and complete.
2	Good attempt. Would you like to try this one again?	Most answers are specific and complete. One or two items may be missing or incomplete.
1	Let's be sure that you understand. I recommend that you try this again. See me for more explanation.	Few answers are specific or complete.

From *Physical Education Assessment Toolkit* by Liz Giles-Brown, 2006, Champaign, IL: Human Kinetics.

Working to Improve Our Community

Name _____ **Unit** _____

BEFORE YOU START

1. Besides working to improve my personal skills and fitness, I am going to help build our community during this unit by doing quality work, being a respectful and responsible class member, and using time efficiently.

2. I will do two specific things:

- _____

  _____

- _____

  _____

AFTER YOU FINISH

Reflect on the two goals that you set for yourself at the beginning of the unit. Explain what you did to achieve them. If you do not feel that you achieved them, explain what you could have done differently so that you could have.

_____

_____

_____

_____

_____

_____

Assessment: Your work will be scored according to the criteria in the following rubric. Use this information to self-assess your work before you hand it in.

4	Excellent work! You went above and beyond!	Answers are specific and complete. Artwork, specific examples, or details that support answers are included.
3	Good work. Everything is here!	Answers are specific and complete.
2	Good attempt. Would you like to try this one again?	Most answers are specific and complete. One or two items may be missing or incomplete.
1	Let's be sure that you understand. I recommend that you try this again. See me for more explanation.	Few answers are specific or complete.

From *Physical Education Assessment Toolkit* by Liz Giles-Brown, 2006, Champaign, IL: Human Kinetics.

Setting Goals and Reflecting

Name _____ Unit _____

BEFORE YOU START

1. During this unit we will be working to improve the following skills: _____
   _____
   _____

2. I have planned learning activities that will help you develop the skills that you listed above. I have set the following goal for all students in class to work toward. By the end of the unit you should be able to _____
   _____
   _____

3. On the lines that follow please set one personal goal that you would like to achieve by the end of the unit.

   • By the end of the unit I want to be able to _____
   _____

   • I am setting this goal for myself because _____
   _____

AFTER YOU FINISH

4. T F   I feel that I met my personal goal.

5. One thing that either helped me meet my goal or kept me from meeting my goal is _____
   _____

6. The specific skill that I improved the most during the unit was _____
   _____

7. My evidence is the following: _____
   _____

8. I am proud of myself because during this unit I _____
   _____

9. During the next unit I am going to try to _____
   _____

10. My favorite part of this unit was when we _____
   _____

   because _____

(continued)

Assessment: Your work will be scored according to the criteria in the following rubric. Use this information to self-assess your work before you hand it in.

4	Excellent work! You went above and beyond!	Answers are specific and complete. Artwork, specific examples, or details that support answers are included.
3	Good work. Everything is here!	Answers are specific and complete.
2	Good attempt. Would you like to try this one again?	Most answers are specific and complete. One or two items may be missing or incomplete.
I	Let's be sure that you understand. I recommend that you try this again. See me for more explanation.	Few answers are specific or complete.

From *Physical Education Assessment Toolkit* by Liz Giles-Brown, 2006, Champaign, IL: Human Kinetics.

Unit Reflections I

Name _____ **Unit** _____

1. Two of the skills that we focused on during this unit were _____

   _____

   _____

2. Choose one of the skills that we worked on and list two important skill cues.

   • Skill _____

   • Skill cue _____

   • Skill cue _____

Shade in the bar to the point that represents your work in physical education during this unit:

3. During this unit I did quality work.

never	some of the time	most of the time

4. During this unit I was a respectful and responsible class member.

never	some of the time	most of the time

5. During this unit I used time efficiently.

never	some of the time	most of the time

Assessment: Your work will be scored according to the criteria in the following rubric. Use this information to self-assess your work before you hand it in.

4	Excellent work! You went above and beyond!	Answers are specific and complete. Artwork, specific examples, or details that support answers are included.
3	Good work. Everything is here!	Answers are specific and complete.
2	Good attempt. Would you like to try this one again?	Most answers are specific and complete. One or two items may be missing or incomplete.
1	Let's be sure that you understand. I recommend that you try this again. See me for more explanation.	Few answers are specific or complete.

Unit Reflections 2

Name _____ **Unit** _____

1. During this unit I know that I improved my _____. I know that I improved because I used to _____ and now I _____

_____

_____

_____

2. I think that I need more practice _____. I can tell that I need more practice because _____

_____

3. I think the best part of the unit was when we _____. I think that this was the best part because it was fun. Two things that made it fun were

   •   _____

   •   _____

4. I think that my teacher did a good job when he or she _____

_____

_____

_____

During the next unit I wish that he or she would _____

_____

_____

_____

5. I am proud of myself because during this unit I _____

_____

_____

_____

Assessment: Your work will be scored according to the criteria in the following rubric. Use this information to self-assess your work before you hand it in.

4	Excellent work! You went above and beyond!	Answers are specific and complete. Artwork, specific examples, or details that support answers are included.
3	Good work. Everything is here!	Answers are specific and complete.
2	Good attempt. Would you like to try this one again?	Most answers are specific and complete. One or two items may be missing or incomplete.
1	Let's be sure that you understand. I recommend that you try this again. See me for more explanation.	Few answers are specific or complete.

From *Physical Education Assessment Toolkit* by Liz Giles-Brown, 2006, Champaign, IL: Human Kinetics.

Reflecting on My Work in Physical Education

Name _____ **Unit** _____

Directions: Shade in the bar to the point that represents your work in physical education class during this unit.

1. I gave 100 percent. The quality of my work was outstanding.

never   some of the time   most of the time

```
[                                                                    ]
```

2. I was a respectful and responsible class member.

never   some of the time   most of the time

```
[                                                                    ]
```

3. I used time efficiently.

never   some of the time   most of the time

```
[                                                                    ]
```

4. The skills that we worked on improving during the unit were _____

_____

5. I am proud of myself because during this unit I _____

_____

_____

(continued)

Reflecting on My Work in Physical Education *(continued)*

Assessment: Your work will be scored according to the criteria in the following rubric. Use this information to self-assess your work before you hand it in.

4	Excellent work! You went above and beyond!	Answers are specific and complete. Artwork, specific examples, or details that support answers are included.
3	Good work. Everything is here!	Answers are specific and complete.
2	Good attempt. Would you like to try this one again?	Most answers are specific and complete. One or two items may be missing or incomplete.
1	Let's be sure that you understand. I recommend that you try this again. See me for more explanation.	Few answers are specific or complete.

From *Physical Education Assessment Toolkit* by Liz Giles-Brown, 2006, Champaign, IL: Human Kinetics.

Reflections Quick Check

Name _____ **Unit** _____

Check off the things that were true about you during the past unit.

QUALITY OF MY WORK

_____ I was on task and focused on the skill work.

_____ I worked hard to improve skills.

_____ I persevered and had an "I can" attitude.

One other thing that I did was _____

_____

MY RESPECT AND RESPONSIBILITY

_____ I was a respectful listener.

_____ I gave effort and energy to the tasks.

_____ I supported my classmates when they needed it.

One other thing that I did was _____

_____

MY USE OF TIME

_____ I responded to signals immediately and appropriately.

_____ I carried out directions and transitions quickly and efficiently.

One other thing that I did was _____

Something I would like my teacher to know is _____

_____

_____

Assessment: Your work will be scored according to the criteria in the following rubric. Use this information to self-assess your work before you hand it in.

4	Excellent work! You went above and beyond!	Answers are specific and complete. Artwork, specific examples, or details that support answers are included.
3	Good work. Everything is here!	Answers are specific and complete.
2	Good attempt. Would you like to try this one again?	Most answers are specific and complete. One or two items may be missing or incomplete.
1	Let's be sure that you understand. I recommend that you try this again. See me for more explanation.	Few answers are specific or complete.

On the Move With Motor Skills

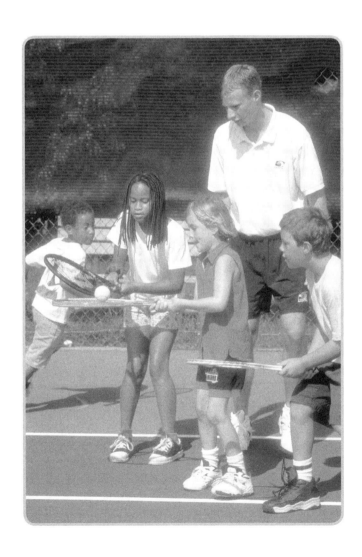

Teaching motor skills is the heart of physical education, the core of everything we do. This chapter provides ideas for using assessment templates that get kids thinking about the mechanics of motor skills, guide them in the self-assessment process, help them objectively assess the performance of others, allow them to apply their knowledge and skills, and track their performance over a given period. All the assessment forms discussed in this chapter are available for reproduction on the accompanying CD-ROM.

The Idea

Helping students improve motor skills at each level is the foundation of most physical education programs. Students need these skills to lead an active lifestyle. This chapter explores the idea of assessing knowledge and understanding of skill cues using self-assessment, peer performance assessments, teacher observation tools, and skill-tracking tasks, with two major objectives in mind:

- To assess learning and make decisions on teaching techniques
- To offer a means by which students can become cognizant of what they can do, what they know, and what they understand

Anybody can get students to move around and play games. The charge of helping students realize their physical abilities and develop a desire to use them outside class is much more difficult. It is not enough for us to assess skills and translate that into a grade on a report card. If we want students to be motivated to use their skills toward developing a healthy and active lifestyle, then we must help them develop confidence in their abilities. We need to offer them opportunities to see their success through positive class experiences and assessment practices.

Assessments

The motor skill assessment templates are designed to be used with any skill being taught. The templates include blank spaces that you can fill in with specific content. You can use most assessments as formative assessments throughout the course of the unit or as summative assessments at the culmination of the unit. The categories of assessments found in this chapter are written assessments,

self-assessments, peer performance assessments, teacher observation tools, skill-tracking tasks, and application tasks.

Written Assessments

Having students write as part of their assessment in physical education has distinct benefits. Writing provides a way for students to communicate what they have learned, allows for interdisciplinary work, provides another way for students to process what they are learning, and can foster creative thinking. The written assessments in this chapter assess the knowledge of skill cues. When considering using written assessments with students, you must recognize that some students will have special needs in this area and may need additional help in completing the task. Communicating with those who provide these children with the services they need is critical. With some students, providing a way to dictate answers may be necessary.

Assessing the knowledge of skill cues is particularly beneficial when skills are new to the learner. At this time, close attention is paid to the movement itself. Skill Cues (form 4.1), Basic Skills (form 4.2), Skill Sentences (form 4.3), Kinesiology (form 4.4), and I'm Just Learning (form 4.5) offer different ways to assess whether students can identify the cues specific to the given skill. The process of writing down these skill cues provides another way in which students can learn and remember them.

The following forms take the notion of getting kids to identify skill cues a step further:

- Imagine That . . . (form 4.6)
- The Alien (form 4.7)
- Hey! I'm Talking to You! (form 4.8)
- Dear Mom, Dad, Grandma, or Grandpa (form 4.9)
- Teach Me! (form 4.10)
- Help Me! Tryouts Are Next Week! (form 4.11)
- Look Closely (form 4.12)
- Magical Sports Equipment (form 4.13)

In these templates students are asked to tap their creative juices in one way or another. To complete these assessments, students must take on a role or use their imagination in some way. Some students enjoy the creative aspect, thus adding a motivational benefit.

Picture It (form 4.14) and You Ought to Be in Pictures! (form 4.15) provide a way in which students can use artwork or photography to show the skill cues for the given skill. Show Me What

You Know—You Choose How! (form 4.16) offers students a variety of ways to complete the assignment and show what they know. All the written assessment templates for motor skills ask for generally the same information; they just go about it in different ways. In chapter 10, Force It—The Alien (form 10.3) is used as a summative assessment during a throwing and catching unit developed for grades three through five. Substituting any of the other assessments would produce the same outcome. Students become bored when they have to do things the same way every time. Having a variety of tools that you can use to bring about the same outcome keeps them thinking. For tips on using these forms, see "Putting It Into Practice: Written Assessments" on page 60.

Self-Assessment

Self-evaluation is a valuable tool for all educators. It teaches kids to think about their learning and their personal performance with objectivity. By thinking about where they are in terms of developing specific skills, students can create a clear vision of where they need to go and what they need to do to move forward. Skill Stages (form 4.17) is a template in which you can fill in any motor skill being focused on during any unit. The first time you use this template, you need to take time to help students understand the three steps of learning a skill. You can role-play different steps and have students practice identifying what stage the learner might be in. Because the template is written in the first person, students can readily identify with one of the stages as they read it. In my experience most students in fifth through eighth grade are accurate when they place themselves in a particular stage. This assessment is useful when you want students to look further into how they learn motor skills and want them to recognize that learning is a process that takes time. Sometimes students believe that if they aren't good at something right away, they never will be. This type of assessment gets them thinking about learning in physical education as an ongoing process. For tips on using this form, see "Putting It Into Practice: Self-Assessment" on page 61.

Peer Performance Assessments

When students do peer assessments they are not only providing valuable information for their fellow students but also going through the mental process of thinking skills through in their own minds. This procedure further cements the information in the brain. In addition, they are learning

what it means to be objective, which is sometimes a hard but important lesson to learn.

Mechanics Check 1 and 2 (forms 4.18 and 4.19) are simple tools to use when you want students to focus on the specific cues outlined for a skill. These two templates are good to use with skills that are important for successful participation in a variety of activities (such as throwing and catching). Although you can fill in skill cues before instruction begins, the effect is more powerful if those cues come from the class, with you acting as a facilitator to be sure that they include all necessary elements.

Generating a list of skill cues with students is a simple process that you can easily do during a closure. For this to be effective, you should do it near the beginning of the unit after students have had a chance to practice the skill that will be focused on. When students participate in generating the list of skill cues, they have ownership in the development process and are more likely to remember the cues. The following list of steps will guide you through the process.

- At the end of class have students face their processing partners (see chapter 9 for details on processing partners). Tell the students that they will be working through a process to come up with four easy-to-remember verbal skill cues for the forearm pass in volleyball (or whatever skill you are focusing on).

- Ask them to come to consensus on one important thing to remember when performing the skill, write their skill cue on a piece of paper, and hand it to you on the way out of class.

- Sometime before the next class period, take the skill cues written by students and list them on a whiteboard or flip chart. Put tally marks next to the cues written by more than one group.

- As students enter the gym for the following class meeting, ask them to read the list of skill cues that the class came up with.

- Just before you begin the lesson, instruct them to think about anything that might be missing as they work during the class period.

- At the close of class, have students stand facing their processing partners. Tell them to look at the list again and to sit down if it looks complete. If they do not believe that the list looks complete, they should remain standing.

- Ask students who are still standing to share what they believe is missing. Facilitate the process of adding to the list anything that might be missing if students do not come up with it right away. Do this by demonstrating the skill and asking students to think about the important things that they see you doing to make the movement efficient.

- When you have the completed list, tell students that they will be responsible for working to perform the skill according to the skill cues listed and that they will be assessed on whether they can perform the skill according to the cues.
- Place the skill cues on the template and copy them for students to use later in the unit.

Accuracy Check (form 4.20) is another type of peer assessment that you can use to focus on specific skills. The previous assessment tools focused on the process of performing a skill. Accuracy Check focuses on how accurate the performance is. This type of assessment is especially useful when accuracy is important to successful participation and when it is relatively easy to judge whether the performance was indeed accurate (for example, tennis strokes, basketball shooting, volleyball hits, and target activities). Students need to be able to watch a peer and judge whether each play of the ball is accurate or inaccurate. The information gathered can then be used with the simple formula provided to calculate the student's percent accuracy. This type of assessment used in combination with other more process-oriented assessments can help students realize the relationship between the process and product of their movement. Someone who is consistently performing the skills correctly will probably have a higher percent accuracy. Reserve this type of assessment for students who have had plenty of opportunity to practice the skills being assessed. For tips on using these forms, see "Putting It Into Practice: Peer Performance Assessment" on page 61.

Teacher Observation Tools

Physical educators spend a lot of time observing and offering feedback to promote learning and improvement. Sometimes it's helpful to have an organized way to keep records of skill development for individual students as well as to provide information regarding the effectiveness of teaching and learning activities. Assessing Student Performance (form 4.21) and Skill Stages—Teacher Assessment (form 4.22) do just that. These forms provide a way in which you can check and keep records of student performance during a class period. By keeping the record sheet on a clipboard, you can readily use it during any class period. For tips on using these forms, see "Putting It Into Practice: Teacher Observation Tools" on page 62.

Skill-Tracking Tasks

Skill-tracking tasks are tools that help students record their own skill performance over a given period. Personal Best Skill Tracking (form 4.23), To 100! (form 4.24), Graduating Numbers (form 4.25), Time Trials (form 4.26), and Group Challenge—Double It (form 4.27) were designed to be easily used in multiple units just by adding new skills. The skills do not have to be filled in ahead of time; the students can add them each time the assessment activity is used.

These assessment templates have four useful features. First, they do not involve competition with others but instead foster competition with oneself to show improvement. They provide a way in which students can attempt to beat previous scores and feel good about their accomplishments. The positive feelings associated with their success are tied to physical activity. Second, once they are copied at the beginning of the year, they can be readily used with other units later on. Alternatively, the same skills can be quickly revisited by pulling that assessment out of the class or student folder. The third wonderful thing about these assessments is that they provide a manageable way to look at skill development and improvement in larger classes. The fourth benefit of choosing this type of assessment to use with a unit is that the assessment is also a practice activity. As students attempt to beat previous scores, they are motivated to practice the skills correctly. During their work, you are free to walk around and offer feedback to help students correct mechanics and reach their goals.

Personal Best Skill Tracking (form 4.23) is used in chapter 11 as part of the assessment options in a badminton unit. In that unit, after being instructed on how to use the template, students use it as a warm-up activity for each lesson. The template promotes efficient use of time because students know exactly what they are going to do on entering the gym. The template can be used with both individual skills and partner skills, and students need not have the same partner each time they work on a skill, although that could be a specification. To 100! (form 4.24) and Graduating Numbers (form 4.25) can be used in the same way.

Time Trials (form 4.26) allows for the assessment of skills under a timed situation. As students become more proficient at a skill they are more likely to be accurate or successful in situations that provide a little more pressure. A time trial is one such situation. You can place any skill on the time trial list. Consider these ideas: How many times can you toss, catch, and clap in one minute? How many baskets can you make from within the basketball key in one minute? How many times can you and a partner throw and catch the lacrosse ball in one minute? How many times can you ski (cross-country) back and forth between two cones in one minute?

Group Challenge—Double It (form 4.27) can be used when you have teams set up to use throughout a unit. This activity provides a challenge for groups to double their score each time they make an attempt. When you couple this with some instruction about how to offer positive, specific instructional feedback to peers to help the group effort, you have a two-for-one situation.

An important lesson for all students is to learn that they can play a role in any given situation. More skilled players can learn to help the group by encouraging and offering feedback to fuel improvement. Less skilled students can learn to receive feedback not as a criticism but as a learning tool that can help them improve. With some careful planning, all students can have a chance to play both roles during a year.

One final thing to remember when using these skill-tracking tasks is that discarding them after each year isn't necessary. If students are in the same building for more than one year, their task sheets can be used again. This method can produce evidence of skill improvement over several years when some of the same skills are revisited. For tips on using these forms, see "Putting It Into Practice: Skill-Tracking Tasks" on page 62.

Application Assessment

One of the most rewarding things to observe as a physical education teacher is a student's ability to take feedback available from the results of his or her movement, process that information, and make changes to improve performance. For some, the thinkers, that process comes naturally. They process the information, break down the movement, and make necessary changes to improve on the next trial. Students who do not possess this ability can be led through activities that will help them discover how to become self-directed learners. Using Feedback to Improve Performance (form 4.28) doubles as a lesson activity and assessment tool. This assessment teaches the process of reading feedback taken from the result of performance and translating that information into changes that can be made to the movement to increase efficiency. You can successfully use this template in any activity that requires accuracy, such as target throwing, Frisbee throwing, golf putting, basket shooting, volleyball serving, badminton serving, tennis serving, archery, and so forth. Using this task with more than one activity during the same

year will help with learning transfer. For tips on using this form, see "Putting It Into Practice: Application Assessment" on page 63.

Setting Up Everyone for Success

To be successful when implementing the assessments in this section, students must have a clear understanding of the vocabulary used. Take time to be sure that students understand the terms, such as *skill cues, feedback, objective, learning, practicing,* and *automatic.* Another important understanding for students to have is that of the learning line, especially when involved in self-evaluation and peer evaluation. Explain to students that we are all on a never-ending learning line in every subject area. Some of us are just beginning the journey; some of us with more experience are located at other points along the line. The important concept to remember here is that although we are all in different places, we all have the ability to move forward. Good assessment will show students their successes and their movement along the line.

Improving performance in various motor skills is similar to learning new spelling words, math concepts, or musical pieces. To improve the likelihood of success for all students, we must foster an environment in which they are not compared to each other but are expected to support each other's differences so that everyone can improve. Continuously using the virtues vocabulary throughout each lesson and holding students accountable to practice those virtues will help create an environment in which everyone moves and everyone learns.

On the pages that follow, you will find lists of ideas for putting each type of assessment form into practice with your students. The lists represent ways in which they have been used before and provide space for you to come up with other ways in which you might use them. Following the "Putting It Into Practice" sections, you will find lesson ideas that target some of the assessments in this chapter. The lessons can be used as written or modified to meet specific needs. The Using Feedback Lesson Sequence on page 63 represents part of a Frisbee unit designed to help students further their knowledge and understanding of force production and learn the basic Frisbee throw. This particular assessment works very well with target skills such as shooting in basketball, golf, archery, and so on. Finally, you will find all of the forms referred to in this chapter. They are also found on the accompanying CD-ROM for easy printing and use.

Summary

Building a strong motor skill foundation plays an incredibly important role in the success of children in physical education classes as well as in other activity pursuits. Children need to have many opportunities to practice and develop motor skills in developmentally appropriate activities. The methods chosen to assess skills must also be developmentally appropriate if they are to help strengthen students' knowledge and understanding. This chapter has presented a wide variety of assessments that will be useful as you modify or design physical education units.

PUTTING IT INTO PRACTICE

Written Assessments

You can implement the following ideas when choosing to use one of these assessments.

- **Homework**—Go over the assignment and send students home with physical education homework. They aren't long, involved assignments, and besides yielding good information from the learner, they provide a way to communicate with parents some of the learning that is taking place in physical education.

- **Alone and then with another or others**—Have students fill in the information on their own and then have them share their answers with another student or students. They can discuss their answers and have an opportunity to change or improve on their own.

- **Choices**—Don't we as adults prefer to have choices? Do we like to be told exactly what to do and how to do it? Why not offer choices to our students? We can do that in this situation by choosing two or three templates that will yield essentially the same information and offer students a choice of which one they would like to complete for their assessment. Watch what happens. Just changing the way you present the assignment may profoundly affect students' motivation to complete it.

- **Station option**—When students are working in skill stations, set up one station at which students complete the written assessment. If you have students who have difficulty writing or have special needs in this area, set up a tape recorder so that they can dictate their answers.

- **Ongoing answers**—Give students the assessment template at the beginning of the unit to place in their folders or portfolios. At the end of specific class periods have them get it out and see whether they can complete a portion in a given period.

- **Partner or group work**—Assign partnerships or groups to come to consensus on answers to the questions.

- Other ways in which this type of assessment could be used:

_____

_____

_____

Self-Assessment

▨ **Pre- and postinstruction**—Fill in the skills for the unit and go over the three stages for learning motor skills. Teach the first class of the unit in which you introduce students to the skill cues for the skills and then have them circle the step that they believe they are on at this point. Take time to talk about the steps and what performance in each one looks like. Having students describe a person performing the skill in each stage helps them understand the difference. After the unit is completed, have students return to their assessment and circle where they believe they fall now. Discuss the importance of improvement and what it takes to reach the automatic step.

▨ **Peer assessment**—Have students observe each other during an activity and make a judgment on where they believe their peer falls on the skill stages learning line.

▨ **Adding evidence**—Besides having students do self-assessment on the skill stages, have them choose one of the skills and give specific evidence on the reverse side of the paper as to why they placed themselves in a specific step.

▨ **Station option**—At the end of the unit have students participate in skill stations. Use the self-assessment as one of the stations.

▨ Other ways in which this type of assessment could be used:

_____

_____

_____

Peer Performance Assessment

▨ **One on one**—Students working one on one with a partner during skill practice take turns observing each other.

▨ **Game time**—Students observe a peer participating in a more dynamic activity involving the skill being observed. Partners then change roles.

▨ **Student folders**—Forms can be kept throughout the years spent at a particular school and updated when skills are revisited.

▨ **Skill stations**—As students work in skill stations, you can designate one station as a mechanics check assessment station where students perform a specific task while a partner completes the peer assessment.

▨ Other ways in which this type of assessment could be used:

_____

_____

_____

PUTTING IT INTO PRACTICE

Teacher Observation Tools

- **Pre- and postinstruction**—Before beginning a unit, have students participate in an activity that includes the skill to be observed. Using one of the observation tools, keep a record of their performance. Go through the unit, providing instruction based on what you observed. At the end of the unit, observe students again, making changes on the original observation sheet where needed or using a separate sheet for comparison purposes.
- **Station option**—As students travel through skill stations you can watch those working at the station dedicated to the skill being observed for the day or unit.
- **Ongoing observations**—Use the observation tool to observe two to four students each day during class. Try to look at all students twice during the unit.
- **Videotaped observations**—Set up the videotape to tape either a station or a particular activity in which the skill to be observed is important. Watch the tape after class to record student performance.
- Other ways in which this type of assessment could be used:

_____

_____

_____

PUTTING IT INTO PRACTICE

Skill-Tracking Tasks

- **Warm-up**—After you go over how to use the tracking sheet, students can begin to work as they enter the gym. Students can choose what skill to practice from those listed, or you can choose one to focus on that day.
- **Centers**—You can set up centers that focus on the different skills that students are tracking. Students can choose what skill they would like to work on during a given period.
- **Specific skill work**—As the unit progresses you may find that many students are having difficulty with a specific skill. Add that skill to the list to draw students' focus to that area. Allow additional practice time.
- Other ways in which this type of assessment could be used:

_____

_____

_____

Application Assessment

▧ **Individual assessment**—Partway through the unit, give students instructions according to what the skill is and ask them to complete the assessment on their own.

▧ **Partner activity**—Each student completes his or her own assessment but works with a partner to examine the feedback from two points of view.

▧ **Two activities**—Set up half the space with an application game activity in which students apply the skill. Half the class participates in that activity while the other half completes the assessment. During the following class period the groups switch roles.

▧ Other ways in which this type of assessment could be used:

_____

_____

_____

Using Feedback Lesson Sequence

CONCEPT FOCUS

Feedback, force

SKILL FOCUS

Frisbee throw

EQUIPMENT AND MATERIALS

One Frisbee for each student, materials that students could use to construct a target on the field (cones, dome markers, polyspots, hoops, trash cans), clipboards, pencils, assessment template Using Feedback to Improve Performance (form 4.28)

TEACHING AND LEARNING ACTIVITIES

Step 1: On Target

Warm-Up (5 Minutes)

Students have had previous instruction about stance and delivery and have had opportunities to practice. In this activity, students stand facing each other. One student demonstrates his or her stance and throwing action without releasing the Frisbee but purposely does something wrong. This demonstration will get students thinking about correct mechanics. The other student examines the movement and has two guesses about what is wrong. Students then change roles. After a few minutes have students respond to the question "What goes into a good Frisbee throw?" (Answers might include specifics about grip, stance, release angle, and backswing.)

Target Construction (5 to 10 Minutes)

In this portion of the lesson, students work together to design a target that will be the foundation of the following lessons and the assessment.

Directions

1. Give each partnership 10 minutes to construct a Frisbee target within the designated area.

2. Tell them that they will work at their own target for a while but will also have a chance to work at some of the targets constructed by their classmates. Because they need opportunities to practice throwing different distances, they should not place their target the same distance from the throwing line as any other.

Target Practice (20 to 25 Minutes)

During this activity, students will have a chance to try out the different targets that have been constructed.

Directions

1. Remind students of all the skill cues for grip, stance, and throw. Then have them take turns throwing to their targets.

2. After working at their own targets for a short time, students rotate to the next target on the line and attempt to adjust their delivery to throw to the new target.

3. As they work, ask them to pay close attention to the changes that they make in their throws to come closer to their target.

4. Continue this activity until the class is almost over.

5. Before students pick up their targets, ask them to make mental pictures of their targets so that they can easily reconstruct them for the next class period.

Closure (1 to 2 Minutes)

Processing partners face each other and come to consensus on how to complete the following statement: "Two things I can change to adjust the amount of force that I produce with each throw are . . ."

Step 2: Adjustments

Warm-Up (5 Minutes)

Students move quickly to reconstruct their targets from the day before. When all students have finished they may take a few warm-up throws to their own targets. If flexibility routines are already established, you may want to include them.

Assessment Activity (30 to 35 Minutes)

This activity is a combination class activity and assessment. Students will need most of one class period to complete the assessment.

Directions

1. Call students in and hand out the assessment templates, clipboards, and pencils.

2. Tell them that they are going to use the skills they have developed on how to read what the Frisbee tells them so that they can make adjustments based on the feedback. Tell students to pay close attention to looking at and recording the specifics of where the Frisbee lands each time and the adjustments that they will make as a result of their attempt.

3. Answer any questions and then have partnerships work at their own targets to complete the assessment.

4. If all students complete the assessment before the class period ends, they may rotate to different targets, taking three throws at each one.

Closure (3 to 5 Minutes)

After picking up the targets and handing in their assessments, processing partners face each other and share whether they were able to make the adjustments necessary to increase accuracy.

Note: This assessment is effective with the golf swing or any other target skill.

Skill Cues

Name _____ **Date** _____

Directions: List three important skill cues for _____

_____

1. _____

   _____

   _____

   _____

2. _____

   _____

   _____

   _____

3. _____

   _____

   _____

   _____

Assessment: Your work will be scored according to the criteria in the following rubric. Use this information to self-assess your work before you hand it in.

4	Excellent work! You went above and beyond!	Three correct, complete, specific skill cues are provided. Artwork, specific examples, or details that support answers are included.
3	Good work. Everything is here!	Three correct, complete, specific skill cues are provided.
2	Good attempt. Just a few things are missing. Would you like to give it another try?	At least two of the skill cues provided are correct, complete, and specific.
1	Let's be sure that you understand. I recommend that you try this one again. See me for more explanation.	Fewer than two of the skill cues provided are complete, correct, and specific.

Basic Skills

Name _____ **Date** _____

Directions: A list of basic manipulative skills follows. Next to each skill list three important things that you should focus on when working to further develop that skill. Think of what you have to remember to do to improve and gain consistency. At the end of the year your work will be assessed according to the rubric below. Use a pencil. You will have opportunities to expand on or change your answers.

What do you have to remember when you're learning to be better?

AS A DRIBBLER **1.** _____

2. _____

3. _____

AS A CATCHER **1.** _____

2. _____

3. _____

AS A THROWER **1.** _____

2. _____

3. _____

AS A VOLLEYER **1.** _____

2. _____

3. _____

AS A STRIKER **1.** _____

2. _____

3. _____

AS A TOSSER **1.** _____

2. _____

3. _____

Assessment: Your work will be scored according to the criteria in the following rubric. Use this information to self-assess your work before you hand it in.

4	Excellent work! You went above and beyond!	All the skill cues are correct, complete, and specific for each basic skill. Artwork, specific examples, or details that support answers are included.
3	Good work. Everything is here!	All the skill cues are correct, complete, and specific for each basic skill.
2	Good attempt. Just a few things are missing. Would you like another try?	Most of the skill cues are correct, complete, and specific for each basic skill. Two or three answers may be incorrect, not specific, or incomplete.
1	Let's be sure that you understand. I recommend that you try this one again. See me for more explanation.	Few of the skill cues are correct, complete, and specific for each basic skill.

Skill Sentences

Name _____ **Date** _____

Directions: A skill sentence is a sentence that helps describe an important part of a specific skill. We have been working on the following skills: _____. Use the words listed to the left of each number in complete sentences to describe an important part of each of the skills listed.

_____ 1._____

_____

_____

_____

_____ 2._____

_____

_____

_____

_____ 3._____

_____

_____

_____

_____ 4._____

_____

_____

_____

_____ 5._____

_____

_____

_____

Assessment: Your work will be scored according to the criteria in the following rubric. Use this information to self-assess your work before you hand it in.

4	Excellent work! You went above and beyond!	Each skill sentence describes an important part of the skill listed. Artwork, specific examples, or details that support answers are included.
3	Good work. Everything is here!	Each skill sentence describes an important part of the skill listed.
2	Good attempt. Just a few things are missing. Would you like another try?	At least three of the skill sentences describe an important part of the skill listed.
1	Let's be sure that you understand. I recommend that you try this one again. See me for more explanation.	Fewer than three of the skill sentences describe an important part of the skill listed.

From *Physical Education Assessment Toolkit* by Liz Giles-Brown, 2006, Champaign, IL: Human Kinetics.

FORM 4.4 **Kinesiology**

Name _____ **Date** _____

Directions: Kinesiology is the study of human movement. Studying the actions of the body as it performs different movements can help a learner make adjustments and improvements. Most force-producing movements can be broken down into three distinct parts: preparation, action, and follow-through. Using these three parts, break down _____ by describing what the body does during each part.

Preparation _____

_____

_____

Action _____

_____

_____

Follow-Through _____

_____

_____

TAKE IT FURTHER . . . APPLY YOUR KNOWLEDGE!

Can you think of another skill that has similar movements during each phase? _____

_____

Assessment: Your work will be scored according to the criteria in the following rubric. Use this information to self-assess your work before you hand it in.

4	Excellent work! You went above and beyond!	The answers include accurate descriptions of the body movements in each phase of the skill. Artwork, specific examples, or details that support the answers are included. An additional skill that has similar movements during each phase is provided.
3	Good work. Everything is here!	The answers include accurate descriptions of the movements in each phase of the skill.
2	Good attempt. Just a few things are missing. Would you like to give it another try?	The answers include accurate descriptions of the body movements in two of the phases of the skill.
1	Let's be sure that you understand. I recommend that you try this one again. See me for more explanation.	The answers include accurate descriptions of the body movements in only one or none of the phases of the skill.

From *Physical Education Assessment Toolkit* by Liz Giles-Brown, 2006, Champaign, IL: Human Kinetics.

I'm Just Learning

Name _____ **Date** _____

Directions: While you are learning motor skills you can be thinking about several important things as you practice. The ultimate goal is to be able to perform the skill using correct mechanics without having to think about it at all. In the following thought bubble, write the important skill cues that you need to think about while learning to become more proficient at _____.

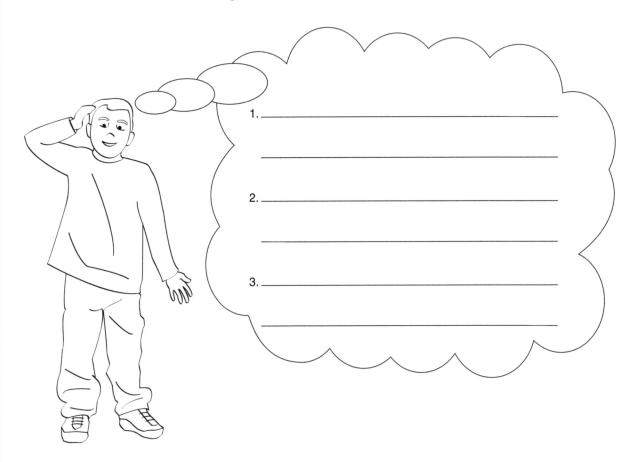

1. _____

_____

2. _____

_____

3. _____

_____

Assessment: Your work will be scored according to the criteria in the following rubric. Use this information to self-assess your work before you hand it in.

4	Excellent work! You went above and beyond!	Three correct, complete, specific skill cues are provided. Artwork, specific examples, or details that support answers are included.
3	Good work. Everything is here!	Three correct, complete, specific skill cues are provided.
2	Good attempt. Just a few things are missing. Would you like to give it another try?	At least two of the skill cues provided are correct, complete, and specific.
1	Let's be sure that you understand. I recommend that you try this one again. See me for more explanation.	Fewer than two of the skill cues provided are complete, correct, and specific.

From *Physical Education Assessment Toolkit* by Liz Giles-Brown, 2006, Champaign, IL: Human Kinetics.

Imagine That . . .

Name _____ **Date** _____

Directions: Imagine that you are a _____

and have been part of physical education class for the past few days. Each day several students use

you as they practice _____. On another piece

of paper, describe a portion of physical education class from your point of view. In your description

you must include how you see students perform _____

_____. Be sure to include all the skill cues (the important things that you should remember

to do) when practicing or performing this skill.

Idea starter: There I was, minding my own business resting in the corner of the huge gymnasium,
when suddenly someone reached down and picked me up.

Assessment: Your work will be scored according to the criteria in the following rubric. Use this
information to self-assess your work before you hand it in.

4	Excellent work! You went above and beyond!	Three correct, complete, specific skill cues are provided in the narrative. Artwork, specific examples, or details that support answers are included.
3	Good work. Everything is here!	Three correct, complete, specific skill cues are provided in the narrative.
2	Good attempt. Just a few things are missing. Would you like to give it another try?	At least two of the skill cues provided in the narrative are correct, complete, and specific.
1	Let's be sure that you understand. I recommend that you try this one again. See me for more explanation.	Fewer than two of the skill cues provided in the narrative are complete, correct, and specific.

From *Physical Education Assessment Toolkit* by Liz Giles-Brown, 2006, Champaign, IL: Human Kinetics.

The Alien

Name _____ **Date** _____

Directions: An alien landed in our gym and watched as we practiced _____. The alien had never seen this skill performed before. The alien noticed, however, that some students were successful and others were having difficulty. What are three things that the alien might have seen the successful students doing that the others were not?

1. _____

_____

_____

_____

2. _____

_____

_____

_____

3. _____

_____

_____

_____

Assessment: Your work will be scored according to the criteria in the following rubric. Use this information to self-assess your work before you hand it in.

4	Excellent work! You went above and beyond!	Three correct, complete, specific skill cues are provided. Artwork, specific examples, or details that support answers are included.
3	Good work. Everything is here!	Three correct, complete, specific skill cues are provided.
2	Good attempt. Just a few things are missing. Would you like to give it another try?	At least two correct, complete, specific skill cues are provided.
1	Let's be sure that you understand. I recommend that you try this one again. See me for more explanation.	Fewer than two complete, correct, specific skill cues are provided.

Hey! I'm Talking to You!

Name _____ **Date** _____

Directions: Poof! The ball that you have been working with has magically acquired human characteristics. The ball can talk, and it has a personality! On a separate piece of paper, write what it might say and how it might say it to help you _____ more successfully. Include at least three pointers.

Assessment: Your work will be scored according to the criteria in the following rubric. Use this information to self-assess your work before you hand it in.

4	Excellent work! You went above and beyond!	Three correct, complete, specific skill cues are provided in the narrative. A strong personality is developed in the narrative that makes the response fun and interesting to read. Artwork, specific examples, or details that support answers are included.
3	Good work. Everything is here!	Three correct, complete, specific skill cues are provided in the narrative.
2	Good attempt. Just a few things are missing. Would you like to give it another try?	At least two of the skill cues provided in the narrative are correct, complete, and specific.
1	Let's be sure that you understand. I recommend that you try this one again. See me for more explanation.	Fewer than two of the skill cues provided in the narrative are complete, correct, and specific.

From *Physical Education Assessment Toolkit* by Liz Giles-Brown, 2006, Champaign, IL: Human Kinetics.

Dear Mom, Dad, Grandma, or Grandpa

Name _____ **Date** _____

Directions: We are currently participating in activities that will help you improve _____.
I bet that some of your family members would be interested in the skills you have been working
to improve in physical education class. Choose a family member to write a note to. Tell him or her
about one of the skills in the following list. In your note, include at least three important skill cues
that you focus on when you practice _____.

_____

_____

_____

_____

_____

_____

_____

_____

_____

_____

_____

_____

Assessment: Your work will be scored according to the criteria in the following rubric. Use this
information to self-assess your work before you hand it in.

4	Excellent work! You went above and beyond!	Three correct, complete, specific skill cues are provided in the letter. Artwork, specific examples, or details that support answers are included.
3	Good work. Everything is here!	Three correct, complete, specific skill cues are provided in the letter.
2	Good attempt. Just a few things are missing. Would you like to give it another try?	At least two of the skill cues provided in the letter are correct, complete, and specific.
1	Let's be sure that you understand. I recommend that you try this one again. See me for more explanation.	Fewer than two of the skill cues provided in the letter are complete, correct, and specific.

Teach Me!

Name _____ **Date** _____

Directions: If you were teaching somebody to _____, you would have to watch him or her and give positive, specific feedback. Write three examples of positive, specific feedback that you could give someone if he or she were doing an excellent job practicing _____.

1. _____

    _____

    _____

    _____

2. _____

    _____

    _____

    _____

3. _____

    _____

    _____

    _____

Assessment: Your work will be scored according to the criteria in the following rubric. Use this information to self-assess your work before you hand it in.

4	Excellent work! You went above and beyond!	All feedback given is positive and specifically refers to key elements of successful performance of the skill. Artwork, specific examples, or details that support answers are included.
3	Good work. Everything is here!	All feedback given is positive and specifically refers to key elements of successful performance of the skill.
2	Good attempt. Would you like to try this one again?	Two examples of the feedback given are positive and specifically refer to key elements of the successful performance of the skill.
1	Let's be sure that you understand. I recommend that you try this one again. See me for more explanation.	Fewer than two examples of the feedback given are positive and specifically refer to key elements of successful performance of the skill.

From *Physical Education Assessment Toolkit* by Liz Giles-Brown, 2006, Champaign, IL: Human Kinetics.

FORM 4.11 **Help Me! Tryouts Are Next Week!**

Name _____ **Date** _____

Directions: Sarah is trying out for the _____ team
and is having difficulty _____. Please help her by
giving three pieces of skill advice that she should focus on to improve her skills and her chances of
making the team.

I. _____

_____

_____

_____

2. _____

_____

_____

_____

3. _____

_____

_____

_____

Assessment: Your work will be scored according to the criteria in the following rubric. Use this
information to self-assess your work before you hand it in.

4	Excellent work! You went above and beyond!	Three correct, complete, specific pieces of skill advice are provided. Artwork, specific examples, or details that support answers are included.
3	Good work. Everything is here!	Three correct, complete, specific pieces of skill advice are provided.
2	Good attempt. Just a few things are missing. Would you like to give it another try?	Two correct, complete, specific pieces of skill advice are provided.
I	Let's be sure that you understand. I recommend that you try this one again. See me for more explanation.	Fewer than two correct, complete, specific pieces of skill advice are provided.

FORM 4.12 **Look Closely**

Name _____ **Date** _____

Directions: Isn't it thrilling to watch how gracefully professional athletes and Olympians move when they perform physical skills? Look closely when you see someone who has mastered the skill of _____. List three things that you notice them doing consistently.

1. _____

   _____

   _____

   _____

2. _____

   _____

   _____

   _____

3. _____

   _____

   _____

   _____

Assessment: Your work will be scored according to the criteria in the following rubric. Use this information to self-assess your work before you hand it in.

4	Excellent work! You went above and beyond!	Three correct, complete, specific skill cues are provided. Artwork, specific examples, or details that support answers are included.
3	Good work. Everything is here!	Three correct, complete, specific skill cues are provided.
2	Good attempt. Just a few things are missing. Would you like to give it another try?	At least two of the skill cues provided are correct, complete, and specific.
1	Let's be sure that you understand. I recommend that you try this one again. See me for more explanation.	Fewer than two of the skill cues provided are complete, correct, and specific.

From *Physical Education Assessment Toolkit* by Liz Giles-Brown, 2006, Champaign, IL: Human Kinetics.

Magical Sports Equipment

Name _____

Directions: Wouldn't it be cool if your sports equipment could communicate with you, giving you pointers and feedback as you participate in different activities? Imagine that you have a magical _____ that you can use whenever you are going to play _____ _____. What's magic about it? Well, it can talk, but only about your performance. It is constantly giving you pointers and tips. You are about to enter a big tournament, and you've been having some problems with your _____. Your magical _____ _____ is about to give you a pep talk. On a separate piece of paper, create the pep talk based on what you know about proper mechanics for this skill. You must include at least three specific pointers. Be creative with this one. Use what you know about voice in your writing. Underline each bit of advice.

Assessment: Your work will be scored according to the criteria in the following rubric. Use this information to self-assess your work before you hand it in.

4	Excellent work! You went above and beyond!	Three correct, complete, specific skill cues are provided in the pep talk. Artwork, specific examples, or details that support answers are included. The sports equipment has been given voice and personality, which makes the response fun to read.
3	Good work. Everything is here!	Three correct, complete, specific skill cues are provided in the pep talk.
2	Good attempt. Just a few things are missing. Would you like to give it another try?	At least two of the skill cues provided in the pep talk are correct, complete, and specific.
1	Let's be sure that you understand. I recommend that you try this one again. See me for more explanation.	Fewer than two of the skill cues provided in the pep talk are complete, correct, and specific.

From *Physical Education Assessment Toolkit* by Liz Giles-Brown, 2006, Champaign, IL: Human Kinetics.

Picture It

Name _____ **Date** _____

Directions: Mental practice is another way to improve performance. It involves picturing yourself performing skills correctly and efficiently. Picture yourself performing the _____ _____. Use drawings or diagrams along with appropriate labels to illustrate yourself performing the correct mechanics for this skill.

Assessment: Your work will be scored according to the criteria in the following rubric. Use this information to self-assess your work before you hand it in.

4	Excellent work! You went above and beyond!	Illustrations depict all the correct mechanics for the specific skill identified in the directions. Labels are appropriate and support the illustrations.
3	Good work. Everything is here!	Illustrations depict most of the correct mechanics for the specific skill identified in the directions. Most of the labels are appropriate and support the illustrations.
2	Good attempt. Just a few things are missing. Would you like to give it another try?	Illustrations depict some of the correct mechanics for the specific skill identified in the directions. Some labels are appropriate and support the illustrations.
1	Let's be sure that you understand. I recommend that you try this one again. See me for more explanation.	Illustrations depict few of the correct mechanics for the specific skill identified in the directions. Labels are inappropriate or missing.

From *Physical Education Assessment Toolkit* by Liz Giles-Brown, 2006, Champaign, IL: Human Kinetics.

You Ought to Be in Pictures!

Name _____ **Date** _____

Directions: Have a friend or family member photograph you with a digital camera performing each part of the _____. Label the important skill cues illustrated by your photographs.

Assessment: Your work will be scored according to the criteria in the following rubric. Use this information to self-assess your work before you hand it in.

4	Excellent work! You went above and beyond!	Photographs depict all the correct mechanics for the specific skill identified in the directions. Labels support the illustrations.
3	Good work. Everything is here!	Photographs depict most of the correct mechanics for the specific skill identified in the directions. Most of the labels support the illustrations.
2	Good attempt. Just a few things are missing. Would you like to give it another try?	Photographs depict some of the correct mechanics for the specific skill identified in the directions. Some labels support the illustrations.
1	Let's be sure that you understand. I recommend that you try this one again. See me for more explanation.	Photographs depict few of the correct mechanics for the specific skill identified in the directions. Labels are inaccurate or missing.

FORM 4.16 **Show Me What You Know— You Choose How!**

Name _____ **Date** _____

Directions: Choose one of the following assignments to complete for the unit. For each assignment you must demonstrate to me that you know the key instructional points or skill cues for _____. These are the skills that we worked on during the unit.

Remember, the purpose of this assignment is for you to show me that you understand how to perform the skills included in the unit and the key instructional points. You must include the skills and instructional points discussed and practiced during the unit.

1. Write a poem that identifies skill cues for the skills that we learned and practiced during this unit.

2. Write a creative story that identifies skill cues for the skills that we learned and practiced during this unit.

3. Design diagrams with skill cues for the skills that we learned and practiced during this unit.

4. Design and write a lesson that you could teach that would educate the participants about skill cues for the skills that we learned and practiced during this unit.

5. Write a dialogue between two people in which one character educates the other about the skill cues for the skills that we learned and practiced during this unit.

6. Design a crossword puzzle that identifies skill cues for the skills that we learned and practiced during this unit. Provide a blank puzzle with the questions (use black or blue ink or the computer). Then copy the puzzle and fill in the correct answers in red ink.

7. Design a skill poster. The poster must be on poster paper and in color. The poster must illustrate and explain skill cues for the skills that we learned and practiced during this unit.

8. Make a collage that identifies skill cues for the skills that we learned and practiced during this unit.

9. Do you have another creative way to demonstrate your knowledge? Discuss it with me for approval.

Assessment: Your work will be scored according to the criteria in the following rubric. Use this information to self-assess your work before you hand it in.

4	Excellent work! You went above and beyond!	Correct, complete, specific skill cues are provided for each skill identified. Artwork, specific examples, or details that support answers are included.
3	Good work. Everything is here!	Most of the project contains correct, complete, specific skill cues for each skill identified.
2	Good attempt. Would you like to try this one again?	Some of the response contains correct, complete, specific skill cues for each skill identified.
1	Let's be sure that you understand. I recommend that you try this one again. See me for more explanation.	Little of the response contains correct, complete, specific skill cues for each skill identified.

Skill Stages

Name _____ **Date** _____

Directions: Read the following stages that a person goes through when learning a skill. Then circle the stage that you feel that you fall in for each skill listed.

Learning stage—I am new to the skill, and my performance is inconsistent. I have to pay close attention to skill cues and think about what I am doing.

Practicing stage—I have mastered the basic mechanics of the skill. I have improved my coordination, control, and consistency.

Automatic stage—My movements have become more automatic and I can use them successfully in a variety of activities. Now I can concentrate on strategy and what is going on around me because I don't have to think about the steps involved in performing the skill.

_____ learning stage   practicing stage   automatic stage

_____ learning stage   practicing stage   automatic stage

_____ learning stage   practicing stage   automatic stage

_____ learning stage   practicing stage   automatic stage

_____ learning stage   practicing stage   automatic stage

_____ learning stage   practicing stage   automatic stage

_____ learning stage   practicing stage   automatic stage

_____ learning stage   practicing stage   automatic stage

_____ learning stage   practicing stage   automatic stage

_____ learning stage   practicing stage   automatic stage

_____ learning stage   practicing stage   automatic stage

_____ learning stage   practicing stage   automatic stage

From *Physical Education Assessment Toolkit* by Liz Giles-Brown, 2006, Champaign, IL: Human Kinetics.

Mechanics Check 1

Skill _____

Performer's Name _____

Assessor's Name _____

Directions: Watch your classmate perform the skill and check the skill cues that you see him or her performing consistently.

☐ **1.** _____
_____

☐ **2.** _____
_____

☐ **3.** _____
_____

Mechanics Check 2

Performer's Name _____

Assessor's Name _____

Directions: Watch your partner as he or she performs the _____.
Pay attention to whether he or she performs the skill cues listed. Shade in the learning line according to your partner's performance.

1. Skill cue _____

never	some of the time	most of the time

2. Skill cue _____

never	some of the time	most of the time

3. Skill cue _____

never	some of the time	most of the time

Accuracy Check

Name of player _____ **Date** _____

Name of scorer _____

Directions: Watch your partner as he or she _____. Each time your partner plays the ball, mark the box according to his or her performance. Place an X in the box if he or she makes an accurate play (ball stays in play, is passed to a teammate, scores, hits the target, or is otherwise successfully played). Mark the box with a 0 if he or she makes an inaccurate play (ball goes out of bounds, doesn't hit the target, is missed, or is otherwise unsuccessfully played).

Total number of plays (X + 0) _____

Formula for percent accuracy: Divide the number of accurate plays (X) by the total number of plays (X + 0). X / (X + 0) = _____ percentage of accurate plays.

FORM 4.21 **Assessing Student Performance**

Date _____ **Grade** _____

Directions: List the four observational cues that you wish to observe. As a student performs, circle or cross out the number corresponding to each cue next to his or her name.

Skill _____

Observational cues   1. _____

2. _____

3. _____

4. _____

_____	1 2 3 4	_____	1 2 3 4	_____	1 2 3 4
_____	1 2 3 4	_____	1 2 3 4	_____	1 2 3 4
_____	1 2 3 4	_____	1 2 3 4	_____	1 2 3 4
_____	1 2 3 4	_____	1 2 3 4	_____	1 2 3 4
_____	1 2 3 4	_____	1 2 3 4	_____	1 2 3 4
_____	1 2 3 4	_____	1 2 3 4	_____	1 2 3 4
_____	1 2 3 4	_____	1 2 3 4	_____	1 2 3 4

From *Physical Education Assessment Toolkit* by Liz Giles-Brown, 2006, Champaign, IL: Human Kinetics.

Skill Stages—Teacher Assessment

Skill _____

Directions: As you observe student performance during class, use this form to record the level at which each student is performing. Write the student's name on the lines under the stage that he or she currently falls into.

AUTOMATIC STAGE

The student is able to demonstrate the skill or skills correctly in isolation.

The student is able to use the skill or skills during practice activities.

The student is able to use the skill or skills during dynamic activities.

_____	_____	_____
_____	_____	_____
_____	_____	_____
_____	_____	_____
_____	_____	_____
_____	_____	_____
_____	_____	_____
_____	_____	_____
_____	_____	_____

PRACTICING STAGE

The student is able to demonstrate the skill or skills correctly in isolation.

The student is able to use the skill or skills during practice activities.

_____	_____	_____
_____	_____	_____
_____	_____	_____
_____	_____	_____
_____	_____	_____
_____	_____	_____
_____	_____	_____
_____	_____	_____

(continued)

From *Physical Education Assessment Toolkit* by Liz Giles-Brown, 2006, Champaign, IL: Human Kinetics.

LEARNING STAGE

The student is able to demonstrate the skill or skills correctly in isolation.

_____   _____   _____

_____   _____   _____

_____   _____   _____

_____   _____   _____

_____   _____   _____

_____   _____   _____

_____   _____   _____

_____   _____   _____

BEGINNING LEARNING STAGE

The student is unable to demonstrate the skill or skills in isolation.

_____   _____   _____

_____   _____   _____

_____   _____   _____

_____   _____   _____

_____   _____   _____

_____   _____   _____

_____   _____   _____

_____   _____   _____

Personal Best Skill Tracking

Name _____ **Grade** _____

Directions: For each skill listed you will be tracking and recording your personal best. Think of it like this: Instead of a book of world records, you have a book of personal records. You must begin again at 1 each time you miss. Write in a new number only if you beat your previous personal best for each skill.

1. _____

2. _____

3. _____

4. _____

5. _____

6. _____

7. _____

8. _____

9. _____

10. _____

To 100!

Name _____ **Grade** _____

Directions: Work alone or with a partner to complete the following tasks. As you work on one of the tasks, shade in the box that contains the numbers that you complete. You may not skip over numbers and must begin at number 1 on each attempt. For example, if you complete three successfully you will shade in the box with the number 3. Then you would work to complete five. You cannot skip from number 3 to number 8. Be sure to do quality skill work, use time efficiently, and be a respectful or responsible classmate.

1. _____

3	5	8	10	15	20	25	30	35	40	50	60	70	80	90	100

2. _____

3	5	8	10	15	20	25	30	35	40	50	60	70	80	90	100

3. _____

3	5	8	10	15	20	25	30	35	40	50	60	70	80	90	100

4. _____

3	5	8	10	15	20	25	30	35	40	50	60	70	80	90	100

5. _____

3	5	8	10	15	20	25	30	35	40	50	60	70	80	90	100

6. _____

3	5	8	10	15	20	25	30	35	40	50	60	70	80	90	100

7. _____

3	5	8	10	15	20	25	30	35	40	50	60	70	80	90	100

8. _____

3	5	8	10	15	20	25	30	35	40	50	60	70	80	90	100

9. _____

3	5	8	10	15	20	25	30	35	40	50	60	70	80	90	100

10. _____

3	5	8	10	15	20	25	30	35	40	50	60	70	80	90	100

Graduating Numbers

Name _____ **Grade** _____

Directions: Graduating numbers is a skill-tracking activity that allows you to work at your own pace. For each skill that you are working to improve, begin counting at number 1. After performing the skill once, you then begin again, attempting to perform the skill two times in a row, under control, without missing. You graduate to the next number only if you successfully complete the number that comes before. In addition, you must always begin at number 1 for each trial. You may not skip any numbers. At the end of the allotted time for this activity, shade over the numbers that you were able to complete with a colored pencil or crayon.

1. Skill _____

1 2 3 4 5 6 7 8 9 10 11 12 13 14 15 16 17 18 19 20 21 22 23 24 25 26 27 28 29 30 31 32 33 34 35 36 37 38 39 40 41 42 43 44 45 46 47 48 49 50 51 52 53 54 55 56 57 58 59 60 61 62 63 64 65 66 67 68 69 70 71 72 73 74 75 76 77 78 79 80 81 82 83 84 85 86 87 88 89 90

2. Skill _____

1 2 3 4 5 6 7 8 9 10 11 12 13 14 15 16 17 18 19 20 21 22 23 24 25 26 27 28 29 30 31 32 33 34 35 36 37 38 39 40 41 42 43 44 45 46 47 48 49 50 51 52 53 54 55 56 57 58 59 60 61 62 63 64 65 66 67 68 69 70 71 72 73 74 75 76 77 78 79 80 81 82 83 84 85 86 87 88 89 90

3. Skill _____

1 2 3 4 5 6 7 8 9 10 11 12 13 14 15 16 17 18 19 20 21 22 23 24 25 26 27 28 29 30 31 32 33 34 35 36 37 38 39 40 41 42 43 44 45 46 47 48 49 50 51 52 53 54 55 56 57 58 59 60 61 62 63 64 65 66 67 68 69 70 71 72 73 74 75 76 77 78 79 80 81 82 83 84 85 86 87 88 89 90

4. Skill _____

1 2 3 4 5 6 7 8 9 10 11 12 13 14 15 16 17 18 19 20 21 22 23 24 25 26 27 28 29 30 31 32 33 34 35 36 37 38 39 40 41 42 43 44 45 46 47 48 49 50 51 52 53 54 55 56 57 58 59 60 61 62 63 64 65 66 67 68 69 70 71 72 73 74 75 76 77 78 79 80 81 82 83 84 85 86 87 88 89 90

5. Skill _____

1 2 3 4 5 6 7 8 9 10 11 12 13 14 15 16 17 18 19 20 21 22 23 24 25 26 27 28 29 30 31 32 33 34 35 36 37 38 39 40 41 42 43 44 45 46 47 48 49 50 51 52 53 54 55 56 57 58 59 60 61 62 63 64 65 66 67 68 69 70 71 72 73 74 75 76 77 78 79 80 81 82 83 84 85 86 87 88 89 90

(continued)

From *Physical Education Assessment Toolkit* by Liz Giles-Brown, 2006, Champaign, IL: Human Kinetics.

6. Skill _____

1 2 3 4 5 6 7 8 9 10 11 12 13 14 15 16 17 18 19 20 21 22 23 24 25 26 27 28 29
30 31 32 33 34 35 36 37 38 39 40 41 42 43 44 45 46 47 48 49 50 51 52 53 54 55
56 57 58 59 60 61 62 63 64 65 66 67 68 69 70 71 72 73 74 75 76 77 78 79 80 81
82 83 84 85 86 87 88 89 90

7. Skill _____

1 2 3 4 5 6 7 8 9 10 11 12 13 14 15 16 17 18 19 20 21 22 23 24 25 26 27 28 29
30 31 32 33 34 35 36 37 38 39 40 41 42 43 44 45 46 47 48 49 50 51 52 53 54 55
56 57 58 59 60 61 62 63 64 65 66 67 68 69 70 71 72 73 74 75 76 77 78 79 80 81
82 83 84 85 86 87 88 89 90

8. Skill _____

1 2 3 4 5 6 7 8 9 10 11 12 13 14 15 16 17 18 19 20 21 22 23 24 25 26 27 28 29
30 31 32 33 34 35 36 37 38 39 40 41 42 43 44 45 46 47 48 49 50 51 52 53 54 55
56 57 58 59 60 61 62 63 64 65 66 67 68 69 70 71 72 73 74 75 76 77 78 79 80 81
82 83 84 85 86 87 88 89 90

9. Skill _____

1 2 3 4 5 6 7 8 9 10 11 12 13 14 15 16 17 18 19 20 21 22 23 24 25 26 27 28 29
30 31 32 33 34 35 36 37 38 39 40 41 42 43 44 45 46 47 48 49 50 51 52 53 54 55
56 57 58 59 60 61 62 63 64 65 66 67 68 69 70 71 72 73 74 75 76 77 78 79 80 81
82 83 84 85 86 87 88 89 90

10. Skill _____

1 2 3 4 5 6 7 8 9 10 11 12 13 14 15 16 17 18 19 20 21 22 23 24 25 26 27 28 29
30 31 32 33 34 35 36 37 38 39 40 41 42 43 44 45 46 47 48 49 50 51 52 53 54 55
56 57 58 59 60 61 62 63 64 65 66 67 68 69 70 71 72 73 74 75 76 77 78 79 80 81
82 83 84 85 86 87 88 89 90

Time Trials

Name _____ **Grade** _____

Directions: Each time trial lasts one minute. You will attempt to perform the skill accurately as many times as you can during the one-minute period. Record your best score in the first box. When you beat your score, record the new score in the next box.

1. _____

2. _____

3. _____

4. _____

5. _____

6. _____

7. _____

8. _____

9. _____

10. _____

Group Challenge—Double It

Group members _____

Directions: As your group completes a task, check off the task in the space provided and move to the next task. Each time you graduate to the next task, the challenge doubles. Good luck. Remember to focus on practicing the virtues that contribute to quality cooperative group work.

Skill	*Task*	
1. _____	Perform 2 in a row	☐
2. _____	Perform 4 in a row	☐
3. _____	Perform 8 in a row	☐
4. _____	Perform 16 in a row	☐
5. _____	Perform 32 in a row	☐
6. _____	Perform 64 in a row	☐
7. _____	Perform 128 in a row	☐

From *Physical Education Assessment Toolkit* by Liz Giles-Brown, 2006, Champaign, IL: Human Kinetics.

Using Feedback to Improve Performance

Name _____ **Date** _____

Directions: When participating in physical activities you will find that you can get excellent feedback from the equipment that you are using, whether the object is a basketball, golf ball, badminton birdie, or tennis ball. If you pay attention to what the object tells you about your movement, you can make adjustments to improve your performance. Self-directed learners improve their skills by practicing and paying close attention to the feedback they get from the results of their movements. This activity will help you develop the skill of observing the result of your movement and making suitable adjustments. By using this method, see how long it takes you to achieve some consistency in your performance.

Skill or task _____

_____

_____

Trial #	Where the ball or object landed (how far off—short, long, left, right)	Adjustments (What will you change about your movement to improve accuracy?)
_____	_____	_____
_____	_____	_____
_____	_____	_____
_____	_____	_____
_____	_____	_____
_____	_____	_____
_____	_____	_____
_____	_____	_____
_____	_____	_____

(continued)

Using Feedback to Improve Performance (continued)

Trial #	Where the ball or object landed (how far off—short, long, left, right)	Adjustments (What will you change about your movement to improve accuracy?)
_____	_____	_____
_____	_____	_____
_____	_____	_____
_____	_____	_____
_____	_____	_____
_____	_____	_____
_____	_____	_____
_____	_____	_____
_____	_____	_____

Assessment: Your work will be scored according to the criteria in the following rubric. Use this information to self-assess your work before you hand it in.

4	Excellent work! You went above and beyond!	All 20 trials were completed, and there was a direct relationship between the result of each trial and the changes made in the next trial. The changes to the movement are specific and easy to understand.
3	Good work. Everything is here!	All 20 trials were completed, and there was a direct relationship between the result of most trials and the changes made in the next trial.
2	Good attempt. Just a few things are missing. Would you like to give it another try?	At least 15 trials were completed, and there was a direct relationship between the result of some trials and the changes made in the next trial.
1	Let's be sure that you understand. I recommend that you try this one again. See me for more explanation.	Fewer than 15 trials were completed, and the relationship between the results of the trials and the changes made in the next trial is vague and difficult to understand.

5 CHAPTER

Concept Connection

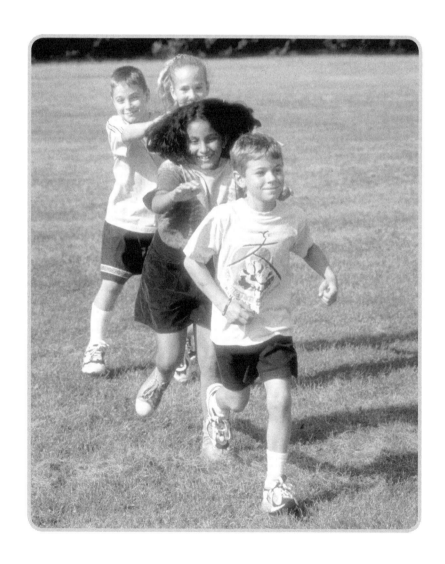

This book would not be complete without a chapter on using assessment to help students make connections between skills and concepts. Most assessments in this chapter are application assessments in which students have opportunities to demonstrate their understanding of movement concepts by completing a movement task. A unique approach to assessing these types of tasks permits students to complete the learning process by making adjustments based on feedback and attempting the task more than once rather than holding them to the outcome of one performance. All the assessment forms discussed in this chapter are available for reproduction on the accompanying CD-ROM.

The Idea

On-task practice in developmentally appropriate learning activities, effective and appropriate feedback, and an understanding of the underlying principles of movement skills will often result in increased learning and skill development. Going beneath the surface of the skills to get students to understand why certain ways of moving are more efficient than others goes beyond teaching for knowledge and delves into teaching for understanding. When students have opportunities to demonstrate their understanding through creative assessment practices designed specifically for that purpose, they will be able to apply what they know to similar skills to improve performance.

Identifying the concepts to focus on during a unit is as important as identifying the skills. Doing this is not always easy. Many of us try to focus on too many concepts during one unit. Chapters 10, 11, and 12 contain three complete units of instruction. Although these units could have included many concepts and principles, they focus on what is most important given the time available, allowing opportunity for experimentation and discovery as well as time to think about how to apply the learning to more than just the skill at hand. For instance, when you teach backspin in relationship to shooting a basketball, you can ask students to think about other skills in which using spin can affect performance or create an advantage. Exploring movement concepts is especially useful in fostering lifelong learning.

Assessments

The assessment templates in this chapter help students demonstrate their understanding of how to apply different concepts to movement to make it more efficient or creative. The assessments fall in two categories—written assessments and application assessments.

Written Assessments

You can use the written assessments in this chapter with any concept that you are teaching. Both Understanding Concepts—Apply It! (form 5.1) and Understanding Concepts—Picture It! (form 5.2) require students to apply their understanding of a specific concept to a specific skill. The concepts and skills to be assessed are up to you. Having students regularly review how understanding the concepts can affect performance is both a powerful teaching tool and a good assessment practice. For tips on using these forms, see "Putting It Into Practice: Written Assessments" on page 100.

Application Assessments

The application assessments take two forms: skill sequences and creative games construction.

Skill Sequence The following assessments all address the understanding and use of movement concepts:

- Locomotor and Axial (Nonlocomotor) Movements (form 5.3)
- Using Space (form 5.4)
- Moving in Different Directions (form 5.5)
- Shapes—Narrow, Wide, Twisted, Round, Symmetrical, and Asymmetrical (form 5.6)
- Using Different Qualities of Time (form 5.7)
- Using Different Qualities of Force (form 5.8)
- Meet, Part, Lead, and Follow (form 5.9)
- Mirrors (form 5.10)
- Unison and Contrast (form 5.11)

You can use these assessments with many different skills. Using skill sequences can serve three purposes:

- To get students to combine the skills that are being focused on during the unit with related concepts

- To give students a chance to demonstrate their understanding of the designated concepts
- To allow for creativity

You can fill in the equipment, movements, or skills that you would like students to build their sequence with, thus allowing for great flexibility. Although the templates in Locomotor and Axial (Nonlocomotor) Movements (form 5.3), Using Space (form 5.4), Moving in Different Directions (form 5.5), Shapes—Narrow, Wide, Twisted, Round, Symmetrical, and Asymmetrical (form 5.6), Using Different Qualities of Time (form 5.7), Using Different Qualities of Force (form 5.8), Meet, Part, Lead, and Follow (form 5.9), Mirrors (form 5.10), and Unison and Contrast (form 5.11) target specific concepts to be worked on, Concepts (form 5.12) leaves space for you to fill in the skills, equipment, and concepts that you want to focus on. For tips on using these forms, see "Putting It Into Practice: Skill Sequence" on page 101.

Creative Games   A creative games assessment is effective when the objective is for students to demonstrate an understanding of the laws that govern their movement and the skills that they have been working to master. For instance, when working on kicking skills, you could ask students to design a game that requires participants to use their kicking skills to create the most amount of force possible. The template Creating Games (form 5.13) allows you to decide what equipment students can use as well as what skills and concepts they are required to apply. For tips on using this form, see "Putting It Into Practice: Creative Games" on page 102.

Setting Up Everyone for Success

Getting students to understand that principles and concepts underlie all movement is not always easy. When students really start thinking about movement in this way, they can begin to think about how much control they have over how they perform.

- Some kids are natural thinkers. They think about the concepts and make changes based on the different types of feedback available.

They are already beginning to be self-directed learners. And isn't that what we want?

- Some students make the same mistakes at the end of the unit that they made when they began. Getting them to slow down and think is sometimes difficult but well worth the effort.

You can do several things to foster this type of learning. The first is to allow time for experimentation and discovery at all ages. As students get older, teachers sometimes skip over the experimentation time because they view it as fooling around or just play. Letting kids experiment with equipment to find out what they can make it do is a great way to start. Second, ask leading questions instead of just telling them how things work. Use lead-ins like "Can you figure out a way to . . ." or "What do you think will happen if we try . . ." By modeling these types of questions, we encourage students to begin asking them of themselves. Another thing that you can do to help students demonstrate lifelong learning habits is to give them a chance to show what they can do or have discovered. Set up times when they can show their peers what they have accomplished. Scheduling this demonstration and combining it with what it means to be a good audience and supportive class member can have a significant influence on students' performance during class.

On the pages that follow, you will find lists of ideas for putting each type of assessment form into practice with your students. The lists represent ways in which they have been used before and provide space for you to come up with other ways in which you might use them. Following the "Putting It Into Practice" sections, you will find lesson ideas that target some of the assessments in this chapter. The lessons can be used as written or modified to meet specific needs. The Magical Mirror Museum Lesson Sequence on page 102 represents part of a unit that includes a skill sequence assessment. The steps outline how to use the assessment after students have been involved in learning activities that include mirroring movements and skills that require mirroring somebody else's movements. The students' goal is to demonstrate understanding of mirroring movements by creating a skill sequence using Mirrors (form 5.10). The movements to be filled in can be any nonlocomotor movements. The Creating Games Lesson Sequence on page

104 represents part of a unit in which a creative games assessment is used. The steps represent the use of the assessment after students have been involved in teaching and learning activities that include foot dribbling using change of speed, direction, and pathway. The target that students are aiming for is to demonstrate understanding of moving an object by using changes of speed, direction, and pathway by using the assessment Creating Games (form 5.13). Blank spaces are provided for you to fill in the equipment available, skills, and concepts. To use this example, you would need to fill in *balls, cones, spots, and hoops* for equipment available, *foot dribbling* for skills, and *using changes of speed, direction, and pathway* for concepts. Finally, you will find all of the forms referred to in this chapter. They are also found on the accompanying CD-ROM for easy printing and use.

Summary

Using the assessments presented in this chapter can further skill development by helping students understand the different ways in which the body can move as well as the concepts and principles that govern movement. The ultimate goal is for students to develop the ability to transfer their knowledge and understanding to similar skills. Helping students develop an understanding of why one way of doing something might be more efficient than another goes beyond just teaching the skills. Students learn to think about the process. When they apply it in the correct way, they move more efficiently. Incorporating some of these assessments into your teaching can have a profound effect on the learning that takes place in your gymnasium, multipurpose room, or playing field.

PUTTING IT INTO PRACTICE

Written Assessments

The number of situations and concepts that you can use with these assessments is almost limitless. Consider the following when deciding what to focus on while teaching different skills.

- **Momentum** (velocity, mass, transfer, sequence, timing)
- **Force** (total force, direction, timing, propelling force, gravity, external force, internal force, friction, muscles, inertia, body levers, resistance, flight, projectile, trajectory, thrust, drag, lift, collision, rebound, spin, elasticity, surface, angle, speed, acceleration)
- **Balance** (stability, gravity, base of support, center of gravity, equilibrium)
- **Health- and skill-related fitness** (cardiorespiratory fitness, endurance, flexibility, muscular strength, muscular endurance, body composition, speed, agility, power, reaction time, movement time, coordination, balance)
- **Strategy** (fake, direction, speed, pathway, vision, peripheral vision, confidence, focus, read position, communication, offense, defense, intent, concealment, space, advantage, repositioning, responsibility, interception, priorities)
- **Information processing** (input, output, external elements, internal elements, decision making, feedback, peripheral field, accuracy, consistency, control, coordination, adaptability, self-directed learning, mental practice)
- **Interactions** (rules, virtues, conflict, communication, consensus, cooperation, competition)
- Other concepts that could be used with this assessment:

_____

_____

_____

Skill Sequence

- **Individual, partner, or group**—Have students design skill sequences alone, with partners, or in small groups. Some students prefer to work by themselves, whereas others might want to do a group skill sequence. In some instances you could give them that choice. Some concepts lend themselves better to individual work, and others work better with partners or small groups.

- **Culminating activity**—After leading students through activities designed to teach the skill and concept focus, use a skill sequence assessment as a culminating activity to include student performance, when you can assess the final product.

- **Videotaped performance**—Videotape the final skill sequence performance and have students do a self-assessment based on the rubric.

- **When you're ready**—Allow students to choose when they would like to be assessed within a certain period. Their job is to design the sequence according to the rubric and then choose a time to be assessed before the deadline. This approach gives them responsibility and allows some choice, which can serve as a motivating factor.

- **If at first**—Allow students to choose when they would like to be assessed but also allow them to be assessed a second time if they want to improve their performance from the first try.

- **Peer assessment day**—Let students know that they must have their sequence completed by a certain class period designated as the assessment day. On that day students may ask other students to do peer assessments. A certain number of assessments can be done, or that choice can be left up to the students based on what they need to improve. Another stipulation might be that they must ask you to do one of the assessments on that day besides those done by their peers. A discussion about objectivity should precede this activity.

- **Set the stage**—Create a situation in which the students place themselves when designing a skill sequence. For instance, if students are working on ball-handling skills and you want them to design a skill sequence that demonstrates understanding of direction, you could set the stage by telling them to imagine that they are part of a professional basketball team that goes around the country performing their skills for many people. Part of the task could be creating a team name. They have been hired to design part of the ball-handling warm-up routine, which must include all skills and concepts included in the rubric. Kids like to pretend and to use their creativity. The sky is the limit when it comes to setting the stage for kids. Just consider what they are interested in and let your imagination take over.

- **Music, music, music**—Choosing the right music can sometimes make a huge difference in designing skills sequences. Letting students have a voice in choosing a piece of music for a given situation is a strong motivator.

- Other ways in which this type of assessment could be used:

_____

_____

_____

Creative Games

■ **As a class**—Before you give this type of assessment to small groups, work through the process as a whole class to design a game that meets the criteria, with you acting as a facilitator. This approach gives students an opportunity to experience the process as it is supposed to be done.

■ **Change a game**—Take a game that the children know well and have them work in groups to change the game to meet the criteria in Creating Games (form 5.13). They may simply have to add skills or concepts to the structure of a game that already exists.

■ **Teach and try**—After students develop their games, you can pair them with other groups to teach each other their games and try to play them. They can then give feedback based on the rubric and offer specific positive comments about the parts that they like.

■ **Book of concept and skill games**—Students who complete the assessment and score a 4 on all items in the rubric can choose to have their game included in a book of games used by the physical education department to help other students develop skills and understand concepts.

■ Other ways in which this type of assessment could be used:

_____

_____

_____

Magical Mirror Museum Lesson Sequence

CONCEPT FOCUS

Mirroring movements

SKILL FOCUS

Nonlocomotor, or axial, movements

EQUIPMENT AND MATERIALS

Mirrors (form 5.10) for each group of students, one pencil for each group, the story about the mirror museum (see step 1), whiteboard, markers, props (optional)

TEACHING AND LEARNING ACTIVITIES

Step 1: Setting the Stage

This step involves setting up kids to begin their skill sequences by taking them through a design process to ensure that everyone can begin the task. Suppose that up to this point students have been working on mirroring movements in many activities and are ready to use them in a skill sequence. Gather students in a circle and tell them the story of the magical mirror museum:

Once upon a time there was a museum full of statues. The statues were made of stone and had been in the museum for hundreds of years. They looked liked normal, everyday statues, posed in many different shapes and levels. But something about these statues was special. Although they could not move they always seemed to have a bit of life, and each statue had an identical twin elsewhere in the museum. When people visited the museum they often commented about having the strange feeling that the statues were watching them. One man in particular loved to visit the museum for the feelings that he had when he was there. He always felt as if he were among real people. One day the man was in a marketplace where an old woman was selling what she claimed to be magic movement powder. The man wondered what would happen if he bought the powder and sprinkled it over the statues that he loved so dearly. He just had to try it. He bought the powder and went directly to the museum. The instant he scattered the powder around the statues, something magical happened. Ever so slightly at first, the powder began to work. The statues started to move, and as they moved, this piece of music played. (Play a piece of slow piano music that will set the stage for slow mirroring movements. As students listen to the music, ask them to close their eyes and imagine what it would feel like to be a statue for so long, unable to move, and then to receive this incredible gift—the gift of movement. Ask them, "What would you feel like? What would you want to do? How would you move?")

Step 2: Brainstorming

During this step in the process students begin by brainstorming ideas that will get them started on their movement sequences.

Directions

1. Assign partners to work together for the remainder of this assessment task. Ask them to sit facing each other and come to consensus about how the statues might feel and what they might do.

2. After a few minutes list the students' responses on chart paper so that you can use the list again. Students will come up with varied responses, and you should record them all.

Step 3: Making Choices

This step involves students in choosing from the larger brainstormed list.

Directions

1. Tell students that they are going to experience what it might be like to be those statues. They are going to become the statues, and their partners will be the identical twins located elsewhere in the museum. With their twins they are going to create a mirroring movement sequence based on the story and the feelings that they listed on the chart paper.

2. Give each partnership a piece of paper and ask them to choose six words from the list the class came up with in step 2. Tell them to choose carefully because the six words will be the basis for their movement sequences.

Step 4: Creating Movements

During step 4 students begin developing movements to go with their word choices.

Directions

1. After each partnership has chosen their words from the list, they begin working on creating movements that show the words.

103

2. Explain that the statues can communicate how they are feeling only through their movements. They cannot talk, but as they come to life they move slowly through the museum until they find their twins. When they find their twins, they seem to know exactly how the other is feeling and they begin to mirror each other's movements. Use an example from their list. Tell students that they are going to design movements to show what the statues might be feeling.

3. Play the music as students work with partners to develop nonlocomotor (axial) mirroring movements that go with each word they chose.

Rarely will all students finish step 4 at the same time.

Step 5: Working on the Sequence

During step 5 students work at their own pace to sequence the movements that they have designed.

Directions

1. As partnerships finish with step 4, give them the assessment Mirrors (form 5.10), with six axial or nonlocomotor movements filled in the blank space designated for skills or movements.

2. You may choose to print the story on the back in case students would like to read it again. Students need to sequence their mirroring movements together with smooth transitions into what you can call their museum sequences.

3. After all students have begun this process, gather them all together at some point and go over the rubric again so that they all know how they will be assessed.

4. As students continue to work you can travel around giving feedback and answering questions.

Step 6: Assessment

Choose a day on which to assess all the sequences. Review the different ways to assess the sequence, listed earlier in this chapter. Choose the method that will work best with your students.

Note: Effective props for this movement sequence are the inexpensive, plain white masks available from mail order catalogues. Partnerships paint twin masks and wear all black clothing to perform their sequences. The props make the situation come to life for the children. Invite another class to watch a final production or have students perform at a school assembly or production.

Creating Games Lesson Sequence

CONCEPT FOCUS

Space, speed, direction, pathway

SKILL FOCUS

Foot dribbling

EQUIPMENT AND MATERIALS

One ball appropriate for foot dribbling and kicking for every student; assorted cones, boundary markers, hoops, or other equipment appropriate for creating games; one Creating Games (form 5.13) assessment sheet for each group of students; one pencil for every student

TEACHING AND LEARNING ACTIVITIES

Step 1: Setting the Stage

This step involves setting up kids to begin creating their game. Taking them through a design process will ensure that everyone can begin the task. Before using this assessment students should have had several opportunities to practice the skills and concepts required. Let students know that during this activity and assessment, they will focus on the concepts of speed, direction, and pathway.

Directions

1. Gather students together and assign them to groups of four. Ask if anyone knows how games are created. (Someone makes them up.) Ask them to list different parts of a game (rules, ways to score, boundaries, jobs, and so on). Talk about how anyone can create a game as long as all players understand how to play and can agree to follow the rules. Then tell them that they are going to create their own foot-dribbling games that will help everyone who plays it practice using changes of speed, direction, and pathway.

2. Take any questions that they might have. Be sure that all students understand the skills and concepts that their games must include. An outside space is best for this activity.

Note that you can use this assessment with many skills and concepts, each having their own space requirements. You need to establish the parameters based on what you want from your students.

Step 2: Brainstorming Games

During this step in the process, students work on coming up with ideas for their games.

Directions

1. Assign groups of students to sit in a circle and brainstorm game ideas. Remind them of the equipment that they may use but emphasize that the game they create is about the skills and concepts, not the equipment. They do not have to use all the equipment, only what they need.

2. Be sure that students know that each person in the group should have the chance to share an idea of what a foot-dribbling game will look like. After each group member has had a chance to share, the group must come to consensus on what game idea they want to use.

3. Tell them to try the game for a few minutes to see how it will work. Remind them to make the best use of their time by practicing good listening and conflict resolution skills.

4. As the groups complete the brainstorming process, they need to move on to the next step. Give them Creating Games (form 5.13) to help them focus on the parts of their game that everyone will need to know.

Step 3: Completing the Assessment Sheet

During this part of the sequence, students work to complete the assessment.

Directions

1. The group first needs to come to consensus on who will be the recorder for the group.

2. After choosing the recorder they should begin working through the sheet, using the consensus decision-making process and making sure that all members of the group have input into answering the questions.

3. Your role at this point is to be a facilitator. Rotate around the space and keep groups on task and moving forward through the process.

Step 4: Game Play

When the groups have finished working through the creative games worksheet, have them try their game again.

Directions

1. Be sure that everyone understands that nothing is engraved in stone. If they feel as if they need to change something as they play the game, they may do so, but they must act as a group.

2. After all groups are engaged in playing their games and have had a good chance to move, stop the action and call all the groups together except one. Tell students that they are going to have a chance to look at all the games that are being developed. Give each group a chance to play their game with the other groups observing.

Note: Taking time for explanations before a group begins is not necessary, and the demonstrations should not take a long time. If an observer has a question about the game, he or she can ask it when you call time. Playing the game and listening to comments and questions from other groups may stimulate groups to make some changes when they go back to work.

Step 5: Assessment

The final step of this process involves a period when each group gets some time to play their game. During this time they can make any changes they wish.

Directions

1. Tell each group that when they feel that their game meets the criteria on the rubric, they should ask you to watch them and do the assessment.

2. After you assess the group's game, go over the completed assessment rubric with them. When working with an assessment like this, you should allow students to make the necessary changes to improve their score if they wish to. After all, the important part of the assessment is not the score, but whether the students learned.

Understanding Concepts—Apply It!

Name _____ **Date** _____

Directions: Explain two ways in which an understanding of the following concept or concepts—
_____—might help you improve

your performance of the following skill or skills: _____.

1. _____

_____

_____

_____

_____

_____

_____

_____

2. _____

_____

_____

_____

_____

_____

_____

Assessment: Your work will be scored according to the criteria in the following rubric. Use this information to self-assess your work before you hand it in.

4	Excellent work! You went above and beyond!	Answers provide two ways in which understanding the concept relates to improved performance of the skill identified. Artwork, specific examples, or details that support answers are included.
3	Good work. Everything is here!	Answers provide two ways in which understanding the concept relates to improved performance of the skill identified.
2	Good attempt. Just a few things are missing. Would you like to give it another try?	Answers provide one way in which understanding the concept relates to improved performance of the skill identified.
1	Let's be sure that you understand. I recommend that you try this one again. See me for more explanation.	Answers fail to provide at least one way in which understanding the concept relates to improved performance of the skill identified.

From *Physical Education Assessment Toolkit* by Liz Giles-Brown, 2006, Champaign, IL: Human Kinetics.

Understanding Concepts—Picture It!

Name _____ **Date** _____

Use drawings or diagrams and labels to illustrate _____.

Assessment: Your work will be scored according to the criteria in the following rubric. Use this information to self-assess your work before you hand it in.

4	Excellent work! You went above and beyond!	The response illustrates the concepts specified in the directions. Labels support the illustrations.
3	Good work. Everything is here!	The response illustrates the concepts specified in the directions. Most of the labels support the illustrations.
2	Good attempt. Just a few things are missing. Would you like to give it another try?	Part of the response illustrates the concepts specified in the directions. Some of the labels support the illustrations.
1	Let's be sure that you understand. I recommend that you try this one again. See me for more explanation.	Little of the response illustrates the concepts specified in the directions. Labels are inaccurate or missing.

From *Physical Education Assessment Toolkit* by Liz Giles-Brown, 2006, Champaign, IL: Human Kinetics.

Locomotor and Axial (Nonlocomotor) Movements

Name _____ **Date** _____

Many concepts can be applied to movement to make it more creative, interesting, challenging, and efficient. In some competitive situations, understanding and applying movement concepts can give you a competitive edge. By completing this assessment you will be able to demonstrate your understanding of the differences between and your ability to perform locomotor skills (gallop, skip, slide, leap) and nonlocomotor skills (twist, sink, rise, bend, stretch, curl, sway).

Directions: Design a movement sequence that meets the criteria for locomotor skills, nonlocomotor skills, and transitions in the following rubric. By using the rubric as you work you can be sure that your sequence will meet or exceed the standard.

Score	Locomotor movements	Nonlocomotor (axial) movements	Transitions
4 Excellent work! You went above and beyond!	Three different locomotor movements are included in the sequence, and they are performed correctly.	Six different nonlocomotor movements are included in the sequence, and they are performed with balance and control.	Transitions between movements in the sequence are smooth. One movement flows without hesitation into the next.
3 Good work. Everything is here!	Two different locomotor movements are included in the sequence, and both are performed correctly.	Four different nonlocomotor movements are included in the sequence, and they are performed with balance and control.	Most transitions between movements are smooth, although slight hesitations occur at times.
2 Good attempt. Just a few things are missing. Would you like another try?	Only one locomotor movement is included in the sequence, and it is performed correctly.	Three different nonlocomotor movements are included in the sequence, and they are performed with balance and control.	Some transitions between movements are smooth. Noticeable hesitations interrupt the flow.
1 Let's be sure that you understand. I recommend that you try this one again. See me for more explanation.	No locomotor movements are included in the sequence, or the locomotor movements included are performed incorrectly.	Only one or two different nonlocomotor movements are included in the sequence, or the nonlocomotor movements are not performed with balance and control.	Few transitions between movements are smooth. Many hesitations interrupt the flow.

From *Physical Education Assessment Toolkit* by Liz Giles-Brown, 2006, Champaign, IL: Human Kinetics.

FORM 5.4 **Using Space**

Name _____ **Date** _____

Many concepts can be applied to movement to make it more creative, interesting, challenging, and efficient. In some competitive situations, understanding and applying movement concepts can give you a competitive edge. By completing this assessment you will be able to demonstrate your understanding of the use of space while practicing the following skills or movements: _____

_____.

Directions: Design a movement sequence that meets the criteria for movements or skills, concepts, and transitions in the following rubric. By using the rubric as you work you can be sure that your sequence will meet or exceed the standard.

Score	Movements or skills	Concept	Transitions
4 Excellent work! You went above and beyond!	All movements or skills identified in the instructions are included in the sequence.	The sequence includes expansive use of general space. Different pathways and levels are included in the sequence.	Transitions between movements in the sequence are smooth. One movement flows without hesitation into another.
3 Good work. Everything is here!	Most of the movements or skills identified in the instructions are included in the sequence.	The sequence includes some use of general space. Different levels are used but movement occurs mostly in straight pathways.	Most transitions between movements are smooth, although slight hesitations occur at times.
2 Good attempt. Just a few things are missing. Would you like another try?	Some of the movements or skills identified in the instructions are included in the sequence.	The sequence includes little use of general space. Most of the movement occurs in personal space with little variation in level.	Some transitions between movements are smooth. Noticeable hesitations interrupt the flow.
1 Let's be sure that you understand. I recommend that you try this one again. See me for more explanation.	Few of the movements or skills identified in the instructions are included in the sequence.	The sequence includes use of personal space only, and movement occurs at only one level.	Few transitions between movements are smooth. Many hesitations interrupt the flow.

From *Physical Education Assessment Toolkit* by Liz Giles-Brown, 2006, Champaign, IL: Human Kinetics.

Moving in Different Directions

Name _____ **Date** _____

Many concepts can be applied to movement to make it more creative, interesting, challenging, and efficient. In some competitive situations, understanding and applying movement concepts can give you a competitive edge. By completing this assessment you will be able to demonstrate your understanding of direction while practicing the following skills or movements: _____

_____.

Directions: Design a movement sequence that meets the criteria for movements or skills, concepts, and transitions in the following rubric. By using the rubric as you work you can be sure that your sequence will meet or exceed the standard.

Score	Movements or skills	Concept	Transitions
4 Excellent work! You went above and beyond!	All movements or skills identified in the instructions are included in the sequence.	All the following directions are included in the sequence: forward, backward, sideways left, sideways right, clockwise, counterclockwise, up, and down.	Transitions between movements in the sequence are smooth. One movement flows without hesitation into another.
3 Good work. Everything is here!	Most of the movements or skills identified in the instructions are included in the sequence.	Six of the following directions are included in the sequence: forward, backward, sideways left, sideways right, clockwise, counterclockwise, up, and down.	Most transitions between movements are smooth, although slight hesitations occur at times.
2 Good attempt. Just a few things are missing. Would you like another try?	Some of the movements or skills identified in the instructions are included in the sequence.	Four of the following directions are included in the sequence: forward, backward, sideways left, sideways right, clockwise, counterclockwise, up, and down.	Some transitions between movements are smooth. Noticeable hesitations interrupt the flow.
1 Let's be sure that you understand. I recommend that you try this one again. See me for more explanation.	Few of the movements or skills identified in the instructions are included in the sequence.	One or two of the following directions are included in the sequence: forward, backward, sideways left, sideways right, clockwise, counterclockwise, up, and down.	Few transitions between movements are smooth. Many hesitations interrupt the flow.

From *Physical Education Assessment Toolkit* by Liz Giles-Brown, 2006, Champaign, IL: Human Kinetics.

Shapes—Narrow, Wide, Twisted, Round, Symmetrical, and Asymmetrical

Name _____ **Date** _____

Many concepts can be applied to movement to make it more creative, interesting, challenging, and efficient. In some competitive situations, understanding and applying movement concepts can give you a competitive edge. By completing this assessment you will be able to demonstrate your understanding of body shapes while practicing the following skills or movements: _____

_____.

Directions: Design a movement sequence that meets the criteria for movements or skills, concepts, and transitions in the following rubric. By using the rubric as you work you can be sure that your sequence will meet or exceed the standard.

Score	Movements or skills	Concept	Transitions
4 Excellent work! You went above and beyond!	All movements or skills identified in the instructions are included in the sequence.	All the following body shapes are included in the sequence: narrow, wide, twisted, round, symmetrical, asymmetrical.	Transitions between movements in the sequence are smooth. One movement flows without hesitation into another.
3 Good work. Everything is here!	Most of the movements or skills identified in the instructions are included in the sequence.	Five of the following six body shapes are included in the sequence: narrow, wide, twisted, round, symmetrical, asymmetrical.	Most transitions between movements are smooth, although slight hesitations occur at times.
2 Good attempt. Just a few things are missing. Would you like another try?	Some of the movements or skills identified in the instructions are included in the sequence.	Three or four of the following six body shapes are included in the sequence: narrow, wide, twisted, round, symmetrical, asymmetrical.	Some transitions between movements are smooth. Noticeable hesitations interrupt the flow.
1 Let's be sure that you understand. I recommend that you try this one again. See me for more explanation.	Few of the movements or skills identified in the instructions are included in the sequence.	One or two of the following six body shapes are included in the sequence: narrow, wide, twisted, round, symmetrical, asymmetrical.	Few transitions between movements are smooth. Many hesitations interrupt the flow.

Using Different Qualities of Time

Name _____ **Date** _____

Many concepts can be applied to movement to make it more creative, interesting, challenging, and efficient. In some competitive situations, understanding and applying movement concepts can give you a competitive edge. By completing this assessment you will be able to demonstrate your understanding of time while practicing the following skills or movements: _____

_____.

Directions: Design a movement sequence that meets the criteria for movements or skills, concepts, and transitions in the following rubric. By using the rubric as you work you can be sure that your sequence will meet or exceed the standard.

Score	Movements or skills	Concept	Transitions
4 Excellent work! You went above and beyond!	All movements or skills identified in the instructions are included in the sequence.	The sequence includes six distinct and subtle changes in the quality of time.	Transitions between movements in the sequence are smooth. One movement flows without hesitation into another.
3 Good work. Everything is here!	Most of the movements or skills identified in the instructions are included in the sequence.	The sequence includes four or five distinct and subtle changes in the quality of time.	Most transitions between movements are smooth, although slight hesitations occur at times.
2 Good attempt. Just a few things are missing. Would you like another try?	Some of the movements or skills identified in the instructions are included in the sequence.	The sequence includes at least three changes in the quality of time.	Some transitions between movements are smooth. Noticeable hesitations interrupt the flow.
1 Let's be sure that you understand. I recommend that you try this one again. See me for more explanation.	Few of the movements or skills identified in the instructions are included in the sequence.	The sequence includes only one or two changes in the quality of time.	Few transitions between movements are smooth. Many hesitations interrupt the flow.

From *Physical Education Assessment Toolkit* by Liz Giles-Brown, 2006, Champaign, IL: Human Kinetics.

Using Different Qualities of Force

Name _____

Many concepts can be applied to movement to make it more creative, interesting, challenging, and efficient. In some competitive situations, understanding and applying movement concepts can give you a competitive edge. By completing this assessment you will be able to demonstrate your understanding of the different qualities of force while practicing the following skills or movements:

_____.

Directions: Design a movement sequence that meets the criteria for movements or skills, concepts, and transitions in the following rubric. By using the rubric as you work you can be sure that your sequence will meet or exceed the standard.

Score	Movements or skills	Concept	Transitions
4 Excellent work! You went above and beyond!	All movements or skills identified in the instructions are included in the sequence.	The sequence includes at least six distinct and subtle changes in the quality of force.	Transitions between movements in the sequence are smooth. One movement flows without hesitation into another.
3 Good work. Everything is here!	Most of the movements or skills identified in the instructions are included in the sequence.	The sequence includes four or five distinct and subtle changes in the quality of force.	Most transitions between movements are smooth, although slight hesitations occur at times.
2 Good attempt. Just a few things are missing. Would you like another try?	Some of the movements or skills identified in the instructions are included in the sequence.	The sequence includes three or four changes in the quality of force.	Some transitions between movements are smooth. Noticeable hesitations interrupt the flow.
1 Let's be sure that you understand. I recommend that you try this one again. See me for more explanation.	Few of the movements or skills identified in the instructions are included in the sequence.	The sequence includes one or two changes in the quality of force.	Few transitions between movements are smooth. Many hesitations interrupt the flow.

From *Physical Education Assessment Toolkit* by Liz Giles-Brown, 2006, Champaign, IL: Human Kinetics.

Meet, Part, Lead, and Follow

Name _____

Many concepts can be applied to movement to make it more creative, interesting, challenging, and efficient. In some competitive situations, understanding and applying movement concepts can give you a competitive edge. By completing this assessment you will be able to demonstrate your understanding of meeting, parting, leading, and following while practicing the following skills or movements:

_____

_____.

Directions: Design a movement sequence that meets the criteria for movements or skills, concepts, and transitions in the following rubric. By using the rubric as you work you can be sure that your sequence will meet or exceed the standard.

Score	Movements or skills	Concept	Transitions
4 Excellent work! You went above and beyond!	All movements or skills identified in the instructions are included in the sequence.	The sequence includes at least three different examples of meeting and parting as well as three different examples of leading and following.	Transitions between movements in the sequence are smooth. One movement flows without hesitation into another.
3 Good work. Everything is here!	Most of the movements or skills identified in the instructions are included in the sequence.	The sequence includes at least two different examples of meeting and parting as well as two different examples of leading and following.	Most transitions between movements are smooth, although slight hesitations occur at times.
2 Good attempt. Just a few things are missing. Would you like another try?	Some of the movements or skills identified in the instructions are included in the sequence.	The sequence includes one example of meeting and parting and one example of leading and following.	Some transitions between movements are smooth. Noticeable hesitations interrupt the flow.
1 Let's be sure that you understand. I recommend that you try this one again. See me for more explanation.	Few of the movements or skills identified in the instructions are included in the sequence.	The sequence includes one example of meeting and parting, or one example of leading and following, or no example of either.	Few transitions between movements are smooth. Many hesitations interrupt the flow.

From *Physical Education Assessment Toolkit* by Liz Giles-Brown, 2006, Champaign, IL: Human Kinetics.

FORM 5.10 **Mirrors**

Name _____

Many concepts can be applied to movement to make it more creative, interesting, challenging, and efficient. In some competitive situations, understanding and applying movement concepts can give you a competitive edge. By completing this assessment you will be able to demonstrate your understanding of mirroring movements while practicing the following skills or movements:

_____ .

Directions: Design a movement sequence that meets the criteria for movements or skills, concepts, and transitions in the following rubric. By using the rubric as you work you can be sure that your sequence will meet or exceed the standard.

Score	Movements or skills	Concept	Transitions
4 Excellent work! You went above and beyond!	All movements or skills identified in the instructions are included in the sequence.	The sequence includes at least six different mirroring movements, and the movers are synchronized throughout the entire sequence.	Transitions between movements in the sequence are smooth. One movement flows without hesitation into another.
3 Good work. Everything is here!	Most of the movements or skills identified in the instructions are included in the sequence.	The sequence includes at least four or five different mirroring movements, and the movers are synchronized for most of the sequence.	Most transitions between movements are smooth, although slight hesitations occur at times.
2 Good attempt. Just a few things are missing. Would you like another try?	Some of the movements or skills identified in the instructions are included in the sequence.	The sequence includes two or three mirroring movements. The movers have difficulty keeping their movements synchronized.	Some transitions between movements are smooth. Noticeable hesitations interrupt the flow.
1 Let's be sure that you understand. I recommend that you try this one again. See me for more explanation.	Few of the movements or skills identified in the instructions are included in the sequence.	The sequence includes one mirroring movement. Little or no synchronization of movements occurs.	Few transitions between movements are smooth. Many hesitations interrupt the flow.

From *Physical Education Assessment Toolkit* by Liz Giles-Brown, 2006, Champaign, IL: Human Kinetics.

Unison and Contrast

Name _____

Many concepts can be applied to movement to make it more creative, interesting, challenging, and efficient. In some competitive situations, understanding and applying movement concepts can give you a competitive edge. By completing this assessment you will be able to demonstrate your understanding of unison and contrast while practicing the following movements or skills: _____
_____.

Directions: Design a movement sequence that meets the criteria for movements or skills, concepts, and transitions in the following rubric. By using the rubric as you work you can be sure that your sequence will meet or exceed the standard.

Score	Movements or skills	Concept	Transitions
4 Excellent work! You went above and beyond!	All movements or skills identified in the instructions are included in the sequence.	The sequence includes at least three different examples of moving in unison and three different examples of contrasting movements or shapes.	Transitions between movements in the sequence are smooth. One movement flows without hesitation into another.
3 Good work. Everything is here!	Most of the movements or skills identified in the instructions are included in the sequence.	The sequence includes at least two different examples of moving in unison and two different examples of contrasting movements or shapes.	Most transitions between movements are smooth, although slight hesitations occur at times.
2 Good attempt. Just a few things are missing. Would you like another try?	Some of the movements or skills identified in the instructions are included in the sequence.	The sequence includes at least one example of moving in unison and one example of contrasting movements or shapes.	Some transitions between movements are smooth. Noticeable hesitations interrupt the flow.
1 Let's be sure that you understand. I recommend that you try this one again. See me for more explanation.	Few of the movements or skills identified in the instructions are included in the sequence.	The sequence includes one example of moving in unison, or one example of a contrasting movement or shape, or no example of either.	Few transitions between movements are smooth. Many hesitations interrupt the flow.

From *Physical Education Assessment Toolkit* by Liz Giles-Brown, 2006, Champaign, IL: Human Kinetics.

Concepts

Name _____

Many concepts can be applied to movement to make it more creative, interesting, challenging, and efficient. In some competitive situations, understanding and applying movement concepts can give you a competitive edge. By completing this assessment you will be able to demonstrate your understanding of _____ while practicing the following movements or skills: _____.

Directions: Design a movement sequence that meets the criteria for movements or skills, concepts, and transitions in the following rubric. By using the rubric as you work you can be sure that your sequence will meet or exceed the standard.

Score	Movements or skills	Concept	Transitions
4 Excellent work! You went above and beyond!	All movements or skills identified in the instructions are included in the sequence.		Transitions between movements in the sequence are smooth. One movement flows without hesitation into another.
3 Good work. Everything is here!	Most of the movements or skills identified in the instructions are included in the sequence.		Most transitions between movements are smooth, although slight hesitations occur at times.
2 Good attempt. Just a few things are missing. Would you like another try?	Some of the movements or skills identified in the instructions are included in the sequence.		Some transitions between movements are smooth. Noticeable hesitations interrupt the flow.
1 Let's be sure that you understand. I recommend that you try this one again. See me for more explanation.	Few of the movements or skills identified in the instructions are included in the sequence.		Few transitions between movements are smooth. Many hesitations interrupt the flow.

From *Physical Education Assessment Toolkit* by Liz Giles-Brown, 2006, Champaign, IL: Human Kinetics.

FORM 5.13 **Creating Games**

Name _____

Many concepts can be applied to motor skills to make movement more efficient. Understanding and applying these concepts can help you be more successful as you perform different motor skills. Your assignment is to use this worksheet with your partners to create a game in which the players must use the following equipment, skills, and concepts:

Equipment available: _____

Skills: _____

Concepts: _____

1. In cooperative games the whole group works together to achieve a goal. In competitive games one team or person tries to outplay or outscore the other team or person. Is your game cooperative or competitive? _____

2. All games have an objective. An objective is simply what the players are trying to do. For example, in basketball the objective is for the players to score baskets by shooting the ball through the hoop while preventing the other team from doing the same. What is the objective for the players in your game?

   _____

   _____

   _____

3. All games have rules. Rules help keep the game organized, safe, and fair. For example, in basketball one rule is that you may not run with the ball. If you move with the ball, you must dribble. If you don't dribble when moving with the ball, the ball is awarded to the other team. What are three important rules in your game?

   A. _____

   B. _____

   C. _____

4. List the skills a person must use in order to participate in your game. _____

   _____

   _____

   _____

(continued)

From *Physical Education Assessment Toolkit* by Liz Giles-Brown, 2006, Champaign, IL: Human Kinetics.

5. Part of this assignment is to design a game in which the players must apply the concepts listed in the directions. Describe how players will need to apply those concepts in order to be successful.

_____

_____

_____

6. When you have finished working on your game, it's time to play. As you play the game, you may decide that you need to change some things. Making decisions is a normal part of developing something new. To change something you will need to gather the group and present your ideas. The group must decide what to do. When you feel that your game is going well and you have met all the criteria, ask me to watch you play. I will score your game based on the following rubric.

Score	Worksheet	Skills	Concepts
4 Excellent work! You went above and beyond!	The answers provided on the worksheet are complete and correct. Artwork, specific examples, or details that support answers are included.	To participate in the game, players must use the skills listed in the directions most of the time.	Participants must apply the concepts listed in the directions most of the time to be successful.
3 Good work. Everything is here!	The answers provided on the worksheet are complete and correct.	To participate in the game, players must use the skills listed in the directions some of the time.	Participants must apply the concepts listed in the directions some of the time in order to be successful.
2 Good attempt. Just a few things are missing. Would you like another try?	Most of the answers on the worksheet are complete and correct.	To participate in the game, players must use the skills listed in the directions in a few instances.	Participants must apply the concepts listed in the directions in a few instances to be successful.
1 Let's be sure that you understand. I recommend that you try this one again. See me for more explanation.	Only a few of the answers on the worksheet are complete and correct. Much information is missing.	Participants could participate successfully in the game and not use the skills listed in the directions at all.	The participants do not need to use the skills listed in the directions to be successful in the game.

6

Focus on Fitness

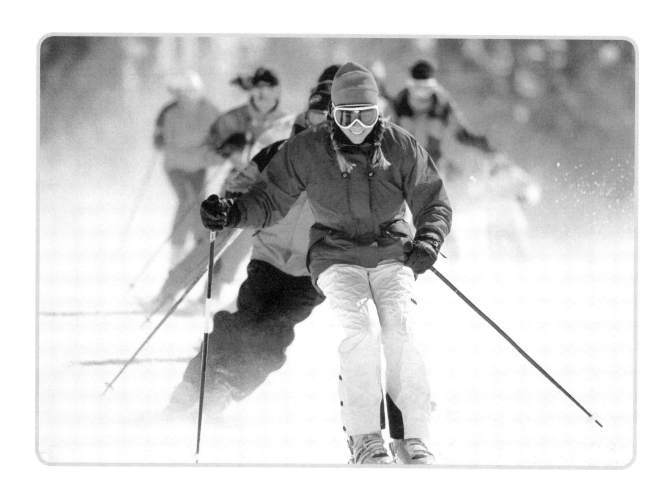

Helping students build fitness knowledge and understanding is the subject of this chapter. In many instances fitness development in physical education programs is difficult to achieve because of time restraints. This chapter is about using the assessment templates to help students develop a strong knowledge base in health- and skill-related fitness so that they can make educated choices about how to focus on fitness and why they should make the effort. All the assessment forms discussed in this chapter are available for reproduction on the accompanying CD-ROM.

The Idea

Traditionally, most physical education programs include a physical fitness unit. The unit allows us to develop lessons that help kids answer the "Why bother?" question. A fitness unit sets time aside to focus on fitness concepts, but it can't end there. Let's take a minute to think about this in another way. What if we took time to thread health- and skill-related fitness concepts into each unit that we teach throughout the year? We would seek to make connections between the parts of fitness that contribute to successful participation in the different activities that we teach.

Wouldn't this approach foster a deeper understanding of the different roles that specific areas of fitness can play throughout a person's life? We can get kids moving in fun activities that attempt to raise heart rates, improve muscular strength and endurance, and increase flexibility. But we should also take time to thread the knowledge and understanding that will motivate and support a person's choices on a day-to-day basis. Using assessments will help us find out whether students understand those relationships. This chapter is dedicated to assessments that address the relationship between health and fitness as well as students' ability to apply fitness concepts to whatever we are teaching during a unit.

Assessments

The categories of assessments found in this chapter are fitness goal setting, testing, and reflecting; knowledge quick-check assessments; application assessments; and out-of-school fitness applications. The knowledge quick-check assessment templates are designed to be used as formative assessments, giving you a chance to assess whether students know basic fitness concepts and vocabulary. The application assessments can be used with any unit. You can fill in the spaces provided with your own content. The out-of-school fitness applications are designed to be used as extra credit that students complete on their own time.

Fitness Goal Setting, Planning, Testing, and Reflecting

Much debate has occurred over the years about fitness testing in physical education classes. Some teachers include it as a part of their regular curriculum, and some do not. Including fitness testing for the sole purpose of testing does not seem like the best use of the limited time available to most physical educators. Combining fitness testing with personal goal setting and reflecting, however, can profoundly affect students' understanding and motivation in this area. Fitness Assessment (form 6.1) is an assessment that you can use for that purpose. You can start this assessment at the beginning of the year, refer to it throughout the year, and then use it again at the end. You can use it with any fitness tests and standards that you choose. After choosing the fitness tests that you will use, fill them in on a blank template and make several copies. The next step is to fill in the standards for girls and boys according to the age and gender of the students that will be participating in the testing. Fill out one template for each and make copies for all students.

Quick Checks for Knowledge

These forms address knowledge of basic health-related fitness concepts and vocabulary and can be used as part of the assessment for a unit that focuses on health-related physical fitness:

- Fitness Quick Check—Health (form 6.2)
- Fitness Quick Check—Components (form 6.3)
- Fitness Quick Check—Risk Factors (form 6.4)
- Fitness Quick Check—Cardio, Cardio, Cardio (form 6.5)
- Fitness Quick Check—Heart Rate (form 6.6)
- Fitness Quick Check—Heart Disease (form 6.7)
- Fitness Quick Check—Warm-Up (form 6.8)
- Fitness Quick Check—Cool-Down (form 6.9)
- Fitness Quick Check—Skill (form 6.10)

- Fitness Quick Check—Vocabulary (form 6.11)
- Fitness Quick Check—Training (form 6.12)

Involving students in activities that contribute positively to their fitness levels is important, of course, but it is equally important for them to be able make the connections between the activities and specific health benefits. The information contained in these assessments creates a basic knowledge base that students can apply later in their lives. When building a unit, you can select these assessments when the desired outcome is for students to be able to demonstrate basic fitness knowledge. The assessments are simple to use and will not take a lot of time for students to complete. For tips on using these forms, see "Putting It Into Practice: Quick Checks for Knowledge" on page 125.

Application Assessments

The application assessments in this chapter provide students with an opportunity to apply their health- and skill-related fitness knowledge to specific situations. Assessments are of two types: written application assessments and performance application assessments. The assessments can be used either within a unit that focuses on health- or skill-related fitness or as a fitness thread for other units that you teach throughout the year. The flexibility of the assessments allows you to add fitness content to any typical skill unit. Giving students a way to take their knowledge a step further and make applications will develop a true understanding of the concepts.

Written Application Assessments The following forms are written application assessments in which students can demonstrate understanding by applying their knowledge of different fitness concepts:

- Apply Your Fitness Knowledge—Amazing Technology (form 6.13)
- Apply Your Fitness Knowledge—You Can Talk? (form 6.14)
- Apply Your Fitness Knowledge—Components (form 6.15)
- Apply Your Fitness Knowledge—Prescribe It (form 6.16)
- Apply Your Fitness Knowledge—Off-Season Training? (form 6.17)
- Apply Your Fitness Knowledge—Fitness Mapping (form 6.18)
- Apply Your Fitness Knowledge—Prescriptions for Good Health (form 6.19)

- Apply Your Fitness Knowledge—Help Me, I Want to Get My Body in Shape! (form 6.20)

Some of these require you to fill in the blank spaces with the content that you want to address. For tips on using these forms, see "Putting It Into Practice: Written Application Assessments" on page 126.

Performance Application Assessments The performance application assessments in this section involve more than writing. These assessments can double as part of the class activity and an assessment. Some writing may be involved, but the focus is on the performance or end product. The details about how to put them into practice are described for each separate assessment.

- **School Fitness Club** In School Fitness Club (form 6.21) students work as a team or class to design a fitness club in the gymnasium using the equipment available in the closet. Students have an opportunity to apply their fitness knowledge to design a club to be used by them or other classes. You can use this assessment as a culminating project during a health-related fitness unit in which the goal is to further students' understanding of the components of health-related fitness. You can use the following lessons as a guide to set this up.
- **Prepractice Routine** Prepractice Warm-Up Routine (form 6.22) can be used to thread fitness into any unit of instruction. This assessment was designed so that students can apply their knowledge of skill-related fitness components, health-related fitness components, and specificity to any activity in order to design sport-specific exercises or activities to use before class begins. After students have completed the assessment, they can use the prepractice routine as they enter class. This assessment is especially effective when you will be dividing the class into teams for the entire unit. Teams can work to complete their prepractice routines with guidance at the beginning of the unit and use them throughout the unit. Teams can also present their routines to other teams so that they learn from each other.
- **Training Sport Specific** Training Sport Specific (form 6.23) works best as a summative assessment after students have had instruction on breaking down activities into their major movements and skill-related fitness components. Either partners or groups

can be used for this assessment. Begin by brainstorming a list of activities that students enjoy participating in. The assessment is more meaningful when students are able to choose the activity that they will focus on because they will choose activities that they enjoy. Try to get students to think outside the box. Do not limit the list to traditional sports. Get them to expand their thinking into a variety of activities. After they brainstorm the list, give them the assessment sheet. Go over the instructions and allow them to use a variety of equipment during their activity selection. Stress that they are training the movements and the skill-related components and that the more creative they are, the more challenging and fun the workout will be. After all students have completed the assignment, have them present their ideas to the rest of the class and assess each person or group using the rubric provided.

- **Get Flexible!** Get Flexible! (form 6.24) is another assessment that you can use to thread fitness concepts into any unit of instruction. The assessment is designed to get students thinking about the muscles used in different activities and how flexibility of those muscles and joints can improve performance. To set up students for this assessment, take a few minutes at the end of the second or third class period to identify the major muscles of the body. Hand out the assessment sheet and go over the instructions. If flexibility has been a normal part of the class routine, students will have an easier time. If it hasn't, they may need some additional instruction. Essentially, their task is to come up with a flexibility exercise that helps prepare the major muscle groups used in the unit activity. They may consult various resources if they need to. On each class meeting after the due date, assign students to present their flexibility exercise by leading the class. One way to assign dates is to put all the dates on slips of paper, place the slips in a hat, and have students draw a date. Assess student work according to the rubric provided.

- **Move It and Improve It!** Move It and Improve It! (form 6.25) is almost the same as Get Flexible! except that the focus is on muscular strength or muscular endurance activities that target the major muscle groups used in the activity for the unit. Therefore, you can follow the same procedure when using this assessment.

Making Connections Outside the Classroom

Nothing is more gratifying to physical educators than to learn that their students are choosing to be active outside school, because they know that their students will not only be having fun but also improving their quality of life. You can use the two templates in this section to get kids thinking more about their activity level outside class. After explaining the program to students and sending an introductory letter to parents in a newsletter, send blank sheets home weekly along with the school newsletter for kids to fill out. Physical Education—Going the Extra Mile! (form 6.26) and Kids in Training for a Healthy and Active Lifestyle (form 6.27) have both been used successfully to get kids to report on physical activity that they do outside class. Whether this program is tied to some extrinsic reward system is up to you. Teachers hold different views on reward systems and how to foster internal motivation. Sometimes the reward is doing something because you know that it's good for you. The body has a neat way of providing its own rewards.

Setting Up Everyone for Success

Some students will be motivated to become physically fit for a grade in physical education, but most will not. People become motivated to make physical activity and fitness a habit when they are involved in positive fitness experiences that teach them the hows and the whys. One person usually cannot make another person fit. Thinking about and making time for physical fitness is a habit that requires understanding the personal benefits associated with that choice.

There are two keys to setting up everyone for success when it comes to teaching physical fitness. The first is making sure that the physical education classroom is safe for all students and that students feel good about themselves when they are there. You must foster an emotionally and physically safe atmosphere where all students are valued for their contributions, where fitness involves personal goal setting instead of competition between class members, and where students feel as though their efforts will not be compared with those of other students. In this environment, students are held accountable for behaving respectfully and responsibly and for practicing the virtues that help to create a positive learning environment.

The second key is to set up teaching, learning, and assessment activities that not only let students experience fitness activities but also help them make the connection between those activities and their personal lives. They need to know why they should bother making the effort to fit fitness into their daily routines.

On the pages that follow, you will find lists of ideas for putting each type of assessment form into practice with your students. The lists represent ways in which they have been used before and provide space for you to come up with other ways in which you might use them. Following the "Putting It Into Practice" sections, you will find lesson ideas that target some of the assessments in this chapter. The lessons can be used as written or modified to meet specific needs. The Fitness Assessment Lesson Sequence on page 126 will help students further their understanding of personal fitness levels. These lessons are not designed to take up an entire class period but instead can be incorporated into a lesson that may be part of the unit that students are currently involved in. The process is worth the time it takes to set up because it can be the foundation for instruction that relates to personal, meaningful goals. The School Fitness Club Lesson Sequence on page 129 is designed as a guide for using the School Fitness Club assessment (form 6.21). Finally, you will find all of the forms referred to in this chapter. They are also found on the accompanying CD-ROM for easy printing and use.

Summary

Pick up any newspaper or magazine and you are almost guaranteed to see something related to physical fitness. You will read reports on inactivity, articles on obesity, and pieces on how to become more physically fit. Wouldn't it be wonderful if all our children learned and practiced fitness habits at an early age so that we wouldn't see so many health problems associated with being inactive? Using the assessments presented in this chapter and threading fitness throughout the curriculum can advance students' knowledge and understanding of health- and skill-related fitness concepts, which we hope will lead them into choosing the habit of fitness over inactivity.

PUTTING IT INTO PRACTICE

Quick Checks for Knowledge

▦ **Closure**—You can use quick checks at the end of a fitness lesson as a vocabulary or concept check.

▦ **Fitness partners**—You can assign fitness partners at the beginning of the unit. As part of the partnership, students come to consensus on what they believe to be the correct answers at the end of a lesson.

▦ **Pre- and postinstruction**—At the beginning of a class, you can use a quick check to get kids thinking about what the lesson will cover. Instruct students to answer the questions before you begin an individual activity. Then, at the end of the lesson, students can revisit their papers and make changes based on the new information they learned.

▦ **Fitness circuit**—Set up a fitness circuit with the assessment sheets as one of the stations.

▦ **Homework**—Students can complete the assessment at home and bring it back to the next class meeting.

▦ Other ways in which this type of assessment could be used:

_____

_____

_____

PUTTING IT INTO PRACTICE

Written Application Assessments

- **Summative assessment**—Use the assessments at the end of a unit as a summative assessment.
- **Ongoing assessment**—Keep assessments in a folder and give them to students at the end of each class period to work on for a given amount of time.
- **Fitness partners**—Assign fitness partners at the beginning of the unit. Give partners time in class to come to consensus on the correct answers and complete the assignment.
- **Homework**—Use the assessment as a homework assignment.
- Other ways in which this type of assessment could be used:

_____

_____

_____

Fitness Assessment Lesson Sequence

CONCEPT FOCUS

Health-related fitness concepts

SKILL FOCUS

Personal goal setting

EQUIPMENT AND MATERIALS

One pencil for every student, one Fitness Assessment (form 6.1) for each student, two index cards for each student, clipboards, brainstorming sheets (see step 2), flip chart or whiteboard, markers, equipment for a variety of fitness stations, fitness-testing equipment necessary for the items chosen for testing, one yellow and one blue marker for each student, and several star stickers per student

TEACHING AND LEARNING ACTIVITIES

Step 1: Getting Started–Setting the Goals

For the introductory lesson you need to have templates filled out with the tests and standards for the ages and number of girls and boys in the class. The focus will be on part I.

Directions

1. After every child has a template and a pencil, begin the class by going over the categories in the table and answering any questions that students might have. Tell students that as part of physical education they will be participating in some personal fitness goal setting, planning, test-

ing, and reflecting. Ask students whether they know what *personal* means. Discuss their answers and tie the discussion to the notion of personal goal setting.

2. Ask students why they think that fitness is a personal subject. Talk about how all people are different and have personal strengths and weaknesses. Spend sufficient time to be sure that students know that a person's fitness levels are personal, that any physical fitness testing they do will not be compared with others but will be measured against set standards, and that their own goals will set the stage for all the fitness work they do.

3. If you have scores from previous years, you will need to help students fill in those scores under the appropriate headings. If scores from previous years are not available, students can leave that section blank, but you will be able to use it during the next year. At this point students have all the information necessary to set their personal goals. Talk about what to consider when setting those goals, particularly the difference between realistic and unrealistic goals.

4. After students have recorded their personal goals, have them write their goals on index cards so that they can readily check them during any class period. You may wish to provide students with two index cards each so that they can keep one at school and one at home.

Note: Placement of this lesson during the year will depend on when the testing is scheduled. Having students set fitness goals and then testing them two weeks later doesn't make much sense. That would be a good way to set up kids to fail. They need time to work toward their goals. If the year starts with the planning and goal setting, students can refer to their goals and plans throughout the year to see how they are progressing. At the close of the year, you can test them so that they can see whether their plans worked.

Step 2: Making the Plan

Students need to know that just setting a goal in life is not enough. They need to have some sort of plan about how to reach it. You need to take time to help students choose activities or exercises that will help them reach their personal fitness goals. The second section of this template addresses that purpose. Space is provided for students to make a cardiorespiratory, flexibility, abdominal strength, and upper-body strength fitness plan. Use this opportunity to see whether students clearly understand the different fitness components. One way to lead students to choose activities or exercises that they might enjoy is to have them brainstorm fitness activities as part of a station activity and then use the lists to choose what to include on their personal plans.

Directions

1. Set up a variety of stations that include activities from each area of fitness. Next to each station place a clipboard and brainstorming sheet with one of the following headings: cardiorespiratory activities, flexibility activities, abdominal strength activities, and upper-body strength activities. The headings on the sheets at each station should correspond with the type of activity being performed at that station. For instance, if one station requires students to jog or power walk, the sheet at that station should have the heading *cardiorespiratory activities.*

2. After students have performed the activity at a station, ask them to take a minute to think about how the activity made them feel, come up with activities or exercises that might make them feel the same way, and list their ideas on the sheet at the station.

3. After work at the stations is complete, take the sheets and gather the students. Compile the lists onto a whiteboard to create a master list that students can refer to in choosing activities for their personal plans.

4. Encourage students to choose activities that they will enjoy participating in so that they will be more likely to follow their plans.

5. Have students fill in the second section of Fitness Assessment (form 6.1) with the activities that they choose to help them reach their personal fitness goals.

Note: From this point on, students simply check their plans periodically during the time leading up to the fitness testing. You can make fitness connections during each physical education class. Doing so requires little time, and continuous reinforcement and application will further students' understanding of the concepts. Chapter 8 discusses using the content posters provided on the accompanying CD-ROM to accomplish this.

Step 3: Testing and Reflecting

You will need to schedule a time to complete fitness testing at some point during the school year. After students complete the testing, they fill in their scores in the appropriate places in the table.

Directions

1. Have students sit by themselves with an assessment form (the focus will be on part I and part III), a yellow marker, a blue marker, and several star stickers. Have students sit by themselves to reflect on their own work; this is not a time to compare and share. Students need to respect one another and focus on their own work.

2. Guide them to figure out whether their scores meet the health fitness standards or fall below them. If they meet the standards, they highlight their scores in yellow. If they fall below the standards, they circle their scores in blue.

3. Next, have students put star stickers next to their new scores if they met their personal goals. Asking the following questions will help them to reflect on their work:
   - "If a person is able to star all his or her scores, what would that tell the person about his or her goal setting?" (The person met all his or her personal fitness goals, the person set realistic goals, the person worked hard to reach his or her goals by following a plan, or the person may have set goals that were too low.)
   - "If a person is unable to star any of his or her scores, what would that tell the person about his or her goal setting?" (The person may have set goals that were too high based on previous scores, or the person didn't follow his or her plan.)

   Note: Students must recognize whether they set realistic or unrealistic goals based on previous scores. The final part of the process is to have students determine whether they need to maintain or improve current fitness levels in each area and make a plan for the future.

4. The first part of part III involves students in thinking about the whole process and identifying something that they can be proud of. Ask volunteers to provide examples. What students write needs to come from within. They might be proud of the hard work that they did to follow their plans, or they may be proud that they ran the mile faster this year than they did last year. They may even take pride in the fact that they encouraged a classmate during the fitness testing or training. Stress that they can focus on whatever they choose and ask them to respond accordingly.

5. The second part of this section involves looking at the scores in relationship to the standards. Based on the information that they have in front of them, students circle whether they need to maintain or improve each part of fitness identified. They then list two things in each area that they can do to maintain or improve their fitness levels. At this point, you collect the papers and check the rubric box that best reflects the work.

This template has been used successfully with students in grades three through eight. After a few years of using this template, students look forward to referring to their old scores and setting and reaching new goals. This paper can go in each student's folder, or you can send it home with the report card along with information on fitness testing and planning.

School Fitness Club Lesson Sequence

CONCEPT FOCUS

Muscular endurance, muscular strength, cardiorespiratory endurance, flexibility

SKILL FOCUS

Various physical skills associated with the stations that students develop, consensus decision making

EQUIPMENT AND MATERIALS

Any physical fitness equipment available for student use, School Fitness Club (form 6.21)

TEACHING AND LEARNING ACTIVITIES

To begin, a decision must be made about how many circuits to set up. You can decide whether you would like each student to be responsible for a station or whether you will assign partners or teams to set up one, two, or maybe three stations. Your decision hinges on whether you want students to practice consensus decision-making skills.

Directions

1. Start by framing the project so that students have a clear picture of what the end product will look like. Tell students that they will be designing their own fitness center at school and will be responsible for being sure that the center provides its members with a well-rounded workout that addresses muscular strength, muscular endurance, cardiorespiratory endurance, and flexibility.

2. Explain that they will have an opportunity to be creative as they choose what activities to include.

3. Hand out the assessment sheets (School Fitness Club, form 6.21) to the individuals or groups and go over the instructions. After students have made their decisions and completed the assignment sheets, collect them and say that you will go over them before the next class meeting.

4. Score the sheets according to the rubric provided and have them ready for the next class meeting. At this point you have two options. You can organize the activities that the students have identified into a circuit or have the students work as a class to complete that task. Your choice will probably depend on how much time is available. If you decide to organize the activities into a circuit, draw a map with the names of the activities and equipment available so that students can begin construction after instructions. If the class is going to design the setup, you will need to facilitate that process based on the activities chosen.

5. During this next class meeting, students can construct the fitness center and then try it. Before the first try, a decision needs to be made about how the center will be run. Will the center operate as a circuit in which everyone does each station and rotates on cue, or can students build a workout based on their individual objectives? The choice will largely depend on the age of the students this assessment is used with.

This project offers an excellent opportunity to involve parents and community members. Wouldn't it be terrific to set up the center designed by the students and have a family fitness night when students could bring in family members for a workout and show off what they have been learning in physical education?

Fitness Assessment

Name _____ **Date** _____

PART I

Fitness test	Fitness component	Previous fitness scores	Fitness standard	Personal goal	Current fitness scores
	Cardiorespiratory endurance				
	Abdominal strength and endurance				
	Flexibility				
	Upper-body strength and endurance				

PART II

Activities that I can do to help me meet my fitness goals

1. My cardiorespiratory fitness plan:

_____

_____

2. My flexibility fitness plan:

_____

_____

3. My upper-body muscular strength and endurance fitness plan:

_____

_____

4. My abdominal muscular strength and endurance fitness plan:

_____

_____

PART III

Looking at the results

- Congratulations! Highlight in yellow all test scores that meet the health standard. Keep up the good work.
- Circle in blue all scores that fall below the health standard. These are fitness areas that you need to work on.
- Congratulations! Place a star next to each of your scores that either met or exceeded your personal goal for that test.

(continued)

Planning ahead for health and fitness

I am proud of myself because this year during our health-related physical fitness work I

_____

_____

_____

Directions: First, circle whether you need to maintain or improve your fitness level in each area. Look closely at your scores in relationship to the standards. Based on your scores, list two things in each fitness area that you can do to maintain or improve your level of fitness.

1. Cardiorespiratory (maintain / improve)

_____

_____

2. Flexibility (maintain / improve)

_____

_____

3. Upper-body strength (maintain / improve)

_____

_____

4. Abdominal strength (maintain / improve)

_____

_____

Assessment: Your work will be scored according to the criteria in the following rubric. Use this information to self-assess your work before you hand it in.

4	Excellent work! You went above and beyond!	Improvement is evident in at least two of the health-related fitness components. Each response is complete and correct. Artwork, specific examples, or details that support answers are included.
3	Good work. Everything is here!	Improvement is evident in at least two of the health-related fitness components. Each response is complete and correct.
2	Good attempt. Just a few things are missing. Would you like to try this one again?	Improvement is evident in at least one of the health-related fitness components. Most responses are complete and correct. One or two items may be missing or incorrect.
1	Let's be sure you understand. I recommend that you try this one again. See me for more explanation.	Improvement is not evident in any of the health-related fitness components. Few complete or correct answers are provided.

Fitness Quick Check—Health

Name _____ **Date** _____

1. What are three components of health-related physical fitness? _____

_____

_____

_____

_____

_____

2. How can having a healthful level of cardiorespiratory fitness positively affect someone's life? _____

_____

_____

_____

_____

_____

3. How can having a healthful level of muscular strength and endurance positively affect someone's life? _____

_____

_____

_____

_____

4. How can having a healthful level of flexibility positively affect someone's life? _____

_____

_____

_____

_____

_____

Scoring: The number of correct answers _____ divided by the number of possible answers _____ equals the percentage of correct answers _____.

From *Physical Education Assessment Toolkit* by Liz Giles-Brown, 2006, Champaign, IL: Human Kinetics.

Fitness Quick Check—Components

Name _____ **Date** _____

1. What are three components of health-related physical fitness? _____

   _____

   _____

   _____

   _____

2. What are three components of skill-related fitness? _____

   _____

   _____

   _____

   _____

Scoring: The number of correct answers _____ divided by the number of possible answers _____ equals the percentage of correct answers _____.

Fitness Quick Check—Risk Factors

Name _____ **Date** _____

1. A risk factor is _____

   _____

   _____

   _____

   _____

2. Three risk factors for heart disease are _____

   _____

   _____

   _____

   _____

Scoring: The number of correct answers _____ divided by the number of possible answers _____ equals the percentage of correct answers _____.

Fitness Quick Check—Cardio, Cardio, Cardio

Name _____ **Date** _____

1. Cardiovascular fitness is _____

2. How long should a cardiorespiratory workout last? _____

3. How many times a week should you do cardiorespiratory activities? _____

4. How hard must you work out during each cardiorespiratory fitness workout? _____

   _____

5. How can you measure the intensity of a cardiovascular workout? _____

6. Name two things that happen to a person's heart when he or she participates regularly in a cardiovascular fitness program.

   1. _____

   2. _____

Scoring: The number of correct answers _____ divided by the number of possible answers _____ equals the percentage of correct answers _____.

Fitness Quick Check—Heart Rate

Name _____ **Date** _____

Person A—This person leads a sedentary lifestyle. He or she is inactive, does not participate in any exercise activities, and makes unhealthful food choices.

Person B—This person is active, chooses to eat a healthful, balanced diet, and participates in regular cardiovascular physical fitness activities.

Persons A and B are about the same age, height, and weight.

1. Who is more likely to have a lower resting heart rate? _____

2. Explain your answer to the previous question. _____

   _____

   _____

   _____

Scoring: The number of correct answers _____ divided by the number of possible answers _____ equals the percentage of correct answers _____.

Fitness Quick Check—Heart Disease

Name _____ **Date** _____

Directions: Use the words provided to fill in the blank spaces.

1. Two common types of heart disease are _____ and _____.

2. Atherosclerosis is caused by deposits of _____ on the artery walls.

3. People who exercise regularly may lower their risk of having a _____ when they are older.

4. People who participate in cardiorespiratory exercise regularly have a _____ heart muscle that is less likely to have problems in the future.

5. People who exercise regularly tend to have a _____ heart rate when resting.

6. Sometimes people who exercise regularly develop extra _____ in their heart.

7. Regular exercise reduces the _____ of heart disease.

atherosclerosis	high blood pressure	fat	strong
heart attack	arteries	lower	risk

Scoring: The number of correct answers _____ divided by the number of possible answers _____ equals the percentage of correct answers _____.

Fitness Quick Check—Warm-Up

Name _____ **Date** _____

1. List one benefit of incorporating a warm-up into a practice or workout.

   _____

2. Give two examples of warm-up activities. _____

   _____

Scoring: The number of correct answers _____ divided by the number of possible answers _____ equals the percentage of correct answers _____.

Fitness Quick Check—Cool-Down

Name _____ **Date** _____

1. List one benefit of incorporating a cool-down into a practice or workout.

   _____

2. Give two examples of possible cool-down activities.

   _____

   _____

Scoring: The number of correct answers _____ divided by the number of possible answers _____ equals the percentage of correct answers _____.

From *Physical Education Assessment Toolkit* by Liz Giles-Brown, 2006, Champaign, IL: Human Kinetics.

Fitness Quick Check—Skill

Name _____ **Date** _____

1. List five components of skill-related fitness.

   _____

   _____

   _____

2. What is one benefit of learning about skill-related fitness components?

   _____

   _____

Scoring: The number of correct answers _____ divided by the number of possible answers _____ equals the percentage of correct answers _____.

From *Physical Education Assessment Toolkit* by Liz Giles-Brown, 2006, Champaign, IL: Human Kinetics.

Fitness Quick Check—Vocabulary

Name _____ **Date** _____

Directions: Match each item with its definition.

_____ **1.** duration   **A.** how often you do something

_____ **2.** frequency   **B.** how long you do something

_____ **3.** intensity   **C.** a measure of how hard you work

Scoring: The number of correct answers _____ divided by the number of possible answers _____ equals the percentage of correct answers _____.

From *Physical Education Assessment Toolkit* by Liz Giles-Brown, 2006, Champaign, IL: Human Kinetics.

Fitness Quick Check—Training

Name _____ **Date** _____

1. When talking about fitness training, specificity means _____
_____

2. When talking about fitness training, overload means _____
_____

3. When talking about fitness, progression means _____
_____

Scoring: The number of correct answers _____ divided by the number of possible answers _____ equals the percentage of correct answers _____.

From *Physical Education Assessment Toolkit* by Liz Giles-Brown, 2006, Champaign, IL: Human Kinetics.

Apply Your Fitness Knowledge— Amazing Technology

Name _____ **Date** _____

Directions: You are part of a research team that has developed a way to reduce a human being to a size small enough to travel inside a body-pod throughout the human body. You have been selected to make the first trip. Think of the observations that you will make and the research that you will be able to do! Your assignment is to go in and make some specific observations on the changes that take place inside the human body when it is involved in cardiorespiratory activity. You will need to describe what is going on as you communicate with the rest of your research team. The list that follows includes a number of items that the team would like you to report on. Next to each item provide a description of what is going on. Use descriptive language to describe what you see.

Heart rate (rate at which the heart beats) _____

_____

_____

_____

Blood flow _____

_____

_____

_____

Stroke volume (amount of blood pumped with each beat of the heart) _____

_____

_____

_____

Assessment: Your work will be scored according to the criteria in the following rubric. Use this information to self-assess your work before you hand it in.

4	Excellent work! You went above and beyond!	Each response is complete and correct. The student was able to identify specific changes that occur in heart rate, blood flow, and stroke volume during exercise. Artwork, specific examples, or details that support answers are included.
3	Good work. Everything is here!	Each response is complete and correct. The student was able to identify specific changes that occur in heart rate, blood flow, and stroke volume during exercise.
2	Good attempt. Just a few things are missing. Would you like to try this one again?	Most responses are complete and correct. One or two items may be missing. The student was able to identify some changes that occur in heart rate, blood flow, and stroke volume during exercise.
1	Let's be sure that you understand. I recommend that you try this one again. See me for more explanation.	Few answers are complete and correct. The student was able to identify few changes that occur in heart rate, blood flow, and stroke volume during exercise.

From *Physical Education Assessment Toolkit* by Liz Giles-Brown, 2006, Champaign, IL: Human Kinetics.

Apply Your Fitness Knowledge— You Can Talk?

Name _____ **Date** _____

Directions: Wouldn't it be neat if the inside parts of your body could communicate with you verbally? Just imagine what your body might tell you! Imagine that your _____ has received this magical gift and will be able to speak, but only for a brief period. It really wants to share with you some of the things that you should keep doing to keep it healthy. Think carefully. What would your _____ say to you if it could give you feedback on two positive things that you do or could be doing regularly to keep it healthy? Be creative and persuasive as you give the human characteristic of speech and personality to an otherwise inanimate body part.

1. _____

_____

_____

_____

_____

_____

_____

2. _____

_____

_____

_____

_____

_____

Assessment: Your work will be scored according to the criteria in the following rubric. Use this information to self-assess your work before you hand it in.

4	Excellent work! You went above and beyond!	Each response is complete and correct. Two appropriate health habits related to the specified body part were identified. Artwork, specific examples, or details that support answers are included.
3	Good work. Everything is here!	Each response is complete and correct. Two appropriate health habits related to the specified body part were identified.
2	Good attempt. Just a few things are missing. Would you like to try this one again?	Most responses are complete and correct. One health habit related to the specified body part was identified.
1	Let's be sure that you understand. I recommend that you try this one again. See me for more explanation.	Few answers are complete and correct. No health habits related to the specified body part were identified.

From *Physical Education Assessment Toolkit* by Liz Giles-Brown, 2006, Champaign, IL: Human Kinetics.

FORM 6.15 **Apply Your Fitness Knowledge— Components**

Name _____ **Date** _____

Directions: All physical activities require specific combinations of health-related fitness components and skill-related fitness components. Choose the two major health-related fitness components for _____ and explain how having high levels of these components will help participants be more successful.

1. _____

   _____

   _____

   _____

   _____

   _____

   _____

   _____

2. _____

   _____

   _____

   _____

   _____

   _____

   _____

   _____

Assessment: Your work will be scored according to the criteria in the following rubric. Use this information to self-assess your work before you hand it in.

4	Excellent work! You went above and beyond!	Each response is complete and correct. Two health-related fitness components are identified, and their relationships to the specified activity are provided. Artwork, specific examples, or details that support answers are included.
3	Good work. Everything is here!	Each response is complete and correct. Two health-related fitness components are identified, and their relationships to the specified activity are provided.
2	Good attempt. Just a few things are missing. Would you like to try this one again?	One response is complete and correct. One health-related fitness component is identified, and its relationship to the specified activity is provided.
1	Let's be sure that you understand. I recommend that you try this one again. See me for more explanation.	No complete and correct answers are provided. No health-related fitness components are identified.

Apply Your Fitness Knowledge— Prescribe It

Name _____ **Date** _____

Directions: Jessie wants to train for _____. Identify two skill-related fitness components that are important for her to develop to be successful in this activity and prescribe one exercise or activity that she can do to help her reach her training goals for each component.

1._____   2._____

_____   _____

_____   _____

_____   _____

_____   _____

_____   _____

_____   _____

_____   _____

_____   _____

_____   _____

_____   _____

_____   _____

_____   _____

Assessment: Your work will be scored according to the criteria in the following rubric. Use this information to self-assess your work before you hand it in.

4	Excellent work! You went above and beyond!	Each response is complete and correct. Two skill-related fitness components are identified, and a prescription for a related training activity for each is provided. Artwork, specific examples, or details that support answers are included.
3	Good work. Everything is here!	Each response is complete and correct. Two skill-related fitness components are identified, and a prescription for a related training activity for each is provided.
2	Good attempt. Just a few things are missing. Would you like to try this one again?	One item is missing or incorrect. One of the two skill-related fitness components identified or a related exercise or activity is incorrect.
1	Let's be sure that you understand. I recommend that you try this one again. See me for more explanation.	No complete and correct answers are provided. Skill-related fitness components or related training activities are incorrect or missing.

FORM 6.17 # Apply Your Fitness Knowledge— Off-Season Training?

Name _____ **Date** _____

Directions: Sam loves to participate in _____. He plays on the school team and goes to special camps in the summer so that he can improve his game play. He is looking for some help in putting together some exercises that he can do when he is unable to participate in his favorite activity. He learned in physical education classes that he should train the specific movements that he uses when participating and that he will need to focus on specific health- and skill-related fitness components. You can help Sam by answering some of the questions that he has asked. Provide your answers in the grid that follows.

1. What are two skill-related fitness components important in my sport?

2. Can you recommend a specific exercise for each of these components that I can include in my training routine?

3. What are two health-related fitness components important in my sport?

4. Can you recommend a specific exercise for each of these components that I can include in my training routine?

Skill-related fitness component _____	Skill-related fitness component _____	Health-related fitness component _____	Health-related fitness component _____
Exercise to target this component _____ _____ _____ _____ _____	Exercise to target this component _____ _____ _____ _____ _____	Exercise to target this component _____ _____ _____ _____ _____	Exercise to target this component _____ _____ _____ _____ _____

Assessment: Your work will be scored according to the criteria in the following rubric. Use this information to self-assess your work before you hand it in.

4	Excellent work! You went above and beyond!	Answers are complete and correct. Two health- and two skill-related fitness components (four total) are identified, and specific exercises that develop each are provided. Artwork, specific examples, or details that support answers are included.
3	Good work. Everything is here!	Answers are complete and correct. Two health-related components and two skill-related fitness components (four total) are identified, and specific exercises that develop each are provided.
2	Good attempt. Just a few things are missing. Would you like to try this one again?	Answers are incomplete. Two components (two health-related components, two skill-related components, or one of each) are identified, and a specific exercise that develops each is provided.
1	Let's be sure that you understand. I recommend that you try this one again. See me for more explanation.	Answers are incomplete. Fewer than two components (either one health-related component, one skill-related component, or neither) are identified. No specific exercises are provided.

**Apply Your Fitness Knowledge—
Fitness Mapping**

Name _____ **Date** _____

HEALTH-RELATED FITNESS AND SKILL-RELATED FITNESS

All physical activities require certain components of health-related fitness (HRF) and skill-related fitness (SRF). Different activities require different combinations of these components. For instance, soccer requires high levels of cardiorespiratory endurance, agility, and coordination. One must be able to last for long periods without getting tired and be able to change direction quickly while moving at top speed when dribbling against defense.

Directions: In the arrow boxes, identify what you believe to be the most important HRF and SRF components that a person needs to possess to be successful while participating in the activity identified in the center square. In the ovals defend your choices by identifying how that component relates to the sport.

Health-related fitness components: cardiorespiratory fitness, muscular strength, muscular endurance, and flexibility

Skill-related fitness components: coordination, agility, power, speed, balance, and reaction time

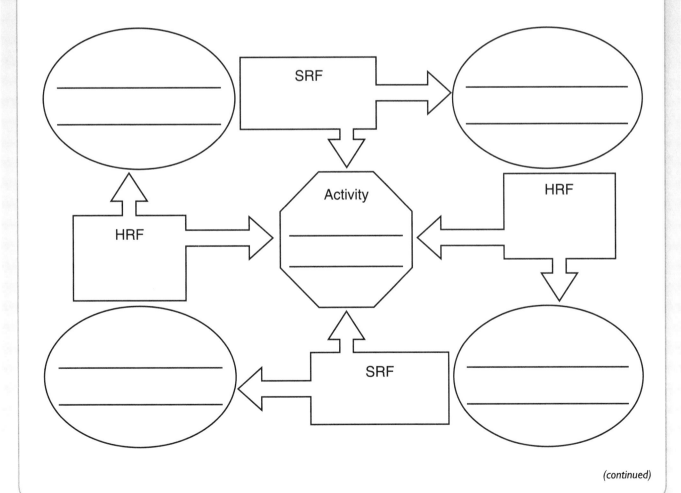

(continued)

From *Physical Education Assessment Toolkit* by Liz Giles-Brown, 2006, Champaign, IL: Human Kinetics.

Apply Your Fitness Knowledge—Fitness Mapping *(continued)*

Assessment: Your work will be scored according to the criteria in the following rubric. Use this information to self-assess your work before you hand it in.

4	Excellent work! You went above and beyond!	Each response is complete and correct. Two health-related fitness components and two skill-related fitness components related to the activity are identified, and a brief explanation of how each relates specifically to the activity is provided. Artwork, specific examples, or details that support answers are included.
3	Good work. Everything is here!	Each response is complete and correct. Two health-related fitness components and two skill-related fitness components related to the activity are identified, and a brief explanation of how each relates specifically to the activity is provided.
2	Good attempt. Just a few things are missing. Would you like to try this one again?	At least two correct health-related or skill-related fitness components (two total) are identified, and a brief explanation of how each relates specifically to the activity is provided.
1	Let's be sure that you understand. I recommend that you try this one again. See me for more explanation.	Fewer than two correct health-related or skill-related fitness components are identified. How they relate to the activity is unclear or missing.

From *Physical Education Assessment Toolkit* by Liz Giles-Brown, 2006, Champaign, IL: Human Kinetics.

Apply Your Fitness Knowledge— Prescriptions for Good Health

Name _____ **Date** _____

Directions: Physicians prescribe many things for people to improve their health. Many are medicines, but some prescriptions are changes in behavior. For this activity you will take on the role of a physician. Your job will be to make prescriptions based on a patient's health-related fitness scores and reported habits. Given the information provided by *one* of the following patients, prescribe activities or exercises that will help the person maintain or improve his or her health-related fitness. Use the prescription sheet provided to make your recommendations. Remember, a person is not likely to engage in activities that he or she does not enjoy, so be sure to consider all the information provided.

PATIENT #3312

Patient #3312 is a 12-year-old boy who just completed some fitness testing. He scored below the health standard for his sex and age in upper-body strength and cardiorespiratory endurance. He met the health standard for abdominal strength and flexibility of the lower back and hamstrings. His nutritional habits include eating mostly sugary cereals and juice for breakfast, school lunch, and a well-balanced supper. He snacks daily on potato chips and soda. His after-school activities include playing video games with his friends and watching television. On weekends he does much of the same.

PATIENT #3313

Patient #3313 is a 13-year-old girl who just completed some fitness testing. She scored below the health standard for her sex and age in upper-body strength and abdominal strength. She met the health standard for cardiorespiratory endurance and flexibility of the lower back and hamstrings. Her nutritional habits include skipping breakfast, eating a bag lunch of mostly fruits, vegetables, and cheese, and eating fast food on the run for dinner because she is part of a busy family. She snacks daily on candy. Her after-school activities include participating in various sports and riding her bike. On weekends she usually has some sporting competition. She also spends some time relaxing with family and friends.

Each Rx (prescription) should include recommendations based on the patient profile. If you include activities, state the number of times or minutes that the patient should perform them (duration) and the number of times per week (frequency). In the rationale section, provide an explanation about why you made this particular prescription. You may also make recommendations about other daily habits that will support a healthy lifestyle.

Fitness Specialists
123 Heart Health Way
Strength, America
304-456-9876

A good fitness plan is one of the best health insurance policies that you can invest in.

(continued)

Apply Your Fitness Knowledge—Prescriptions for Good Health (continued)

Name _____

Rx _____

_____

_____

_____

_____

_____

Rationale

_____

_____

_____

_____

Specialist's signature _____

Assessment: Your work will be scored according to the criteria in the following rubric. Use this information to self-assess your work before you hand it in.

4	Excellent work! You went above and beyond!	Each response is complete and correct. All prescriptions are directly related to the patient profile chosen. A strong rationale is included. Artwork, specific examples, or details that support answers are included.
3	Good work. Everything is here!	Each response is complete and correct. All prescriptions are directly related to the patient profile chosen. A strong rationale is included.
2	Good attempt. Just a few things are missing. Would you like to try this one again?	Most prescriptions made are directly related to the fitness information provided. A rationale is included, but it may not directly relate to the prescriptions. One or two items may be incorrect or missing.
1	Let's be sure that you understand. I recommend that you try this one again. See me for more explanation.	Few complete or correct answers are provided. Most prescriptions do not relate to the patient profile chosen. The rationale is either missing or does not relate to the prescriptions.

Apply Your Fitness Knowledge— Help Me, I Want to Get My Body in Shape!

Name _____ **Date** _____

One of your closest friends has come to you complaining that he or she just doesn't feel that well when participating in physical activities. Your friend says that he or she just can't seem to keep up with everyone else. Your friend really wants to be able to participate in activities without getting tired, strengthen his or her muscles, and not feel so stiff all the time.

Directions: Develop a total fitness poster that will give your friend all the information that he or she needs to achieve his or her goals. Your poster needs to help your friend understand the difference between each fitness component and how to develop each one. Include illustrations to further help him or her understand the concepts.

Your friend needs to know the difference between the following parts of health-related fitness and what activities fall into each category:

_____ Cardiorespiratory fitness

_____ Muscular strength and endurance

_____ Flexibility

You should also include information about the principles of training:

_____ Frequency

_____ Duration

_____ Intensity

Assessment: Your work will be scored according to the criteria listed in the preceding checklist and the rubric below. Use the checklist and rubric to make sure that you have included all the information required on your poster.

4	Excellent work! You went above and beyond!	The poster contains correct, accurate information for all six items identified on the criteria list. Artwork, specific examples, or details that support answers are included.
3	Good work. Everything is here!	The poster contains correct, accurate information for all six items identified on the criteria list.
2	Good attempt. Just a few things are missing. Would you like to try this one again?	The poster contains correct, accurate information for at least four of the six items identified on the criteria list. One or two items may be inaccurate or missing.
1	Let's be sure that you understand. I recommend that you try this one again. See me for more explanation.	The poster contains correct, accurate information for fewer than four of the six items identified on the criteria list.

From *Physical Education Assessment Toolkit* by Liz Giles-Brown, 2006, Champaign, IL: Human Kinetics.

FORM 6.21 **School Fitness Club**

Name _____ **Date** _____

Directions: We are going to create a fitness center in our gymnasium. The fitness center will include activities that improve the following fitness components: _____
_____. Your group is responsible for designing or choosing an activity that meets the requirements for the following fitness categories. Provide all the necessary information for each activity that you choose to include.

Fitness component _____

Activity _____

Equipment needed _____

How will the activity that you choose improve the identified fitness component? _____

_____

_____

_____

Why would you like to include this activity? _____

_____

Fitness component _____

Activity _____

Equipment needed _____

How will the activity that you choose improve the identified fitness component? _____

_____

_____

_____

Why would you like to include this activity? _____

_____

Assessment: Your work will be scored according to the criteria in the following rubric. Use this information to self-assess your work before you hand it in.

4	Excellent work! You went above and beyond!	Activities that support the two specified fitness components are identified, and correct reasons for including them are provided. Artwork, specific examples, or details that support answers are included.
3	Good work. Everything is here!	Activities that support the two specified fitness components are identified, and correct reasons for including them are provided.
2	Good attempt. Just a few things are missing. Would you like to try this one again?	An activity that supports at least one of the specified fitness components is identified, and a correct reason for including it is provided.
1	Let's be sure that you understand. I recommend that you try this one again. See me for more explanation.	Activities and reasons for including them are incorrect.

From *Physical Education Assessment Toolkit* by Liz Giles-Brown, 2006, Champaign, IL: Human Kinetics.

Prepractice Warm-Up Routine

Name _____ **Date** _____

Your team must design a prepractice routine that team members can perform before practice. The routine should help each member further develop two skill-related fitness components and one health-related fitness component specific to _____. Begin by identifying those components in the space provided.

A. Two skill-related fitness components specific to the listed activity are

1. _____   2. _____

B. One health-related fitness component specific to the listed activity is

1. _____

After you have identified the skill- and health-related fitness components, choose three different prepractice exercises or activities that team members can do to improve their performance. On the reverse side of this paper provide names and descriptions for the exercises or activities that you identify and the health- or skill-related fitness components that they target. Team members will use routines at the beginning of each class period. The routines should take about five to eight minutes to complete. Use the following list to be sure that you have met all the criteria.

_____ Two skill-related fitness components and one health-related fitness component specific to the activity are identified.

_____ Three different exercises or activities that target the three skill- and health-related components are identified and explained.

_____ Each team member can perform all exercises or activities.

Assessment: Your work will be scored according to the criteria listed in the preceding checklist and the rubric below. Use the checklist and rubric to make sure that you have included all the items required in your prepractice warm-up.

4	Excellent work! You went above and beyond!	The warm-up meets all the criteria identified. All information related to the warm-up is correct and accurate. Artwork, specific examples, or details that support answers are included.
3	Good work. Everything is here!	The warm-up meets all the criteria identified. All information related to the warm-up is correct and accurate.
2	Good attempt. Just a few things are missing. Would you like to try this one again?	The warm-up meets most of the criteria identified, with most of the information related to the warm-up being correct and accurate. No more than two items are missing or inaccurate.
1	Let's be sure that you understand. I recommend that you try this one again. See me for more explanation.	The warm-up does not meet the criteria identified on the list, and much of the information related to the warm-up is either missing or inaccurate.

FORM 6.23 **Training Sport Specific**

Name _____ **Date** _____

Apply your knowledge of health- and skill-related fitness components.

1. Choose a sport from the class list. _____

2. a. Identify the two major skill-related fitness components and be prepared to defend your choices.

   _____

   _____

   b. Identify one major movement of the sport.

   _____

3. Develop a sequence that trains for the two major skill-related fitness components and the major movement of the sport that you chose from the list. List the sequence of your workout on the back of this paper. You should describe each movement if it does not have a specific name.

4. Prepare a presentation of your sport-specific training sequence.

Assessment: Your work will be scored according to the criteria in the following rubric. Use this information to self-assess your work before you hand it in.

4	Excellent work! You went above and beyond!	The workout includes movements that train the muscles for flexibility and endurance. It also includes movements for the two major skill-related fitness components and the major movements identified. Definite thought went into the design of the workout so that all large muscle movements are grouped to engage the cardiovascular system fully; flexibility exercises and mat exercises were strategically placed for the athlete to get the most benefits from his or her workout. Artwork, specific examples, or details that support answers are included.
3	Good work. Everything is here!	The workout includes movements that train the muscles for flexibility or endurance. It also includes movements for the two major skill-related fitness components and the major movement identified.
2	Good attempt. Just a few things are missing. Would you like to try this one again?	The workout includes movements that train the muscles for flexibility or endurance. It includes movements for one major skill-related fitness component and the major movement identified.
1	Let's be sure that you understand. I recommend that you try this one again. See me for more explanation.	The workout is missing movements that train the muscles for flexibility and endurance. The movements chosen do not train for the skill-related fitness components or the major movement.

FORM 6.24 **Get Flexible!**

Name _____ **Date** _____

Directions: You have been chosen to introduce two new flexibility exercises that will prepare the major muscles used while participating in _____.
We will add these to our normal flexibility routine. You may use resources such as the Internet, books, or exercise professionals. To help you get organized, describe the exercise that you will be presenting on the following lines. Be prepared to lead the class on your assigned date.

1. _____

_____

_____

_____

2. _____

_____

_____

_____

Assessment: Your work will be scored according to the criteria in the following rubric. Use this information to self-assess your work before you hand it in.

4	Excellent work! You went above and beyond!	The two flexibility exercises target major muscle groups used in the specified activity. Artwork, specific examples, or details that support answers are included.
3	Good work. Everything is here!	The two flexibility exercises target major muscle groups used in the specified activity.
2	Good attempt. Just a few things are missing. Would you like to try this one again?	One flexibility exercise targets a major muscle group used in the specified activity. The other either does not target a major muscle group used in the specified activity or is not a flexibility exercise.
1	Let's be sure that you understand. I recommend that you try this one again. See me for more explanation.	Neither flexibility exercise targets major muscle groups used in the specified activity, or the activities presented are not flexibility exercises.

From *Physical Education Assessment Toolkit* by Liz Giles-Brown, 2006, Champaign, IL: Human Kinetics.

FORM 6.25 **Move It and Improve It!**

Name _____ **Date** _____

Directions: Muscular endurance is an important component of many physical activities. Having healthful levels can improve performance. You have been chosen to introduce two new muscular endurance exercises that will target the major muscles used while participating in _____ _____. To help you get organized, describe the activities that you will be presenting on the following lines. Be prepared to lead the class on your assigned date.

1. _____

   _____

   _____

   _____

2. _____

   _____

   _____

   _____

Assessment: Your work will be scored according to the criteria in the following rubric. Use this information to self-assess your work before you hand it in.

4	Excellent work! You went above and beyond!	The muscular strength or endurance exercises target major muscle groups used in the specified activity. Artwork, specific examples, or details that support answers are included.
3	Good work. Everything is here!	The muscular endurance exercises target major muscle groups used in the specified activity.
2	Good attempt. Just a few things are missing. Would you like to try this one again?	One muscular endurance exercise targets a major muscle group used in the specified activity. The other either does not target a major muscle group used in the specified activity or is not a muscular endurance exercise.
1	Let's be sure that you understand. I recommend that you try this one again. See me for more explanation.	Neither muscular endurance exercise targets major muscle groups used in the specified activity, or the activities presented are not muscular endurance exercises.

**Physical Education—
Going the Extra Mile!**

Directions: Fill out a card, cut it out, sign it, have your parent or guardian sign it, and turn it in to your physical education teacher. Each completed card will count as extra credit in physical education.

— —

I WENT THE EXTRA MILE!

Name _____ **Date** _____
—

   1. Name the activity or exercise that you did. _____

   2. How long did you exercise or how many did you do? _____

   3. What category of fitness does this activity or exercise fall under? (circle one)

      A. cardiorespiratory   B. muscular strength and endurance   C. flexibility

_____   _____

Student signature — — — — — — —   Parent or guardian signature — — — — —

I WENT THE EXTRA MILE!

Name _____ **Date** _____
—

   1. Name the activity or exercise that you did. _____

   2. How long did you exercise or how many did you do? _____

   3. What category of fitness does this activity or exercise fall under? (circle one)

      A. cardiorespiratory   B. muscular strength and endurance   C. flexibility

_____   _____

Student signature — — — — — — —   Parent or guardian signature — — — — —

I WENT THE EXTRA MILE!

Name _____ **Date** _____
—

   1. Name the activity or exercise that you did. _____

   2. How long did you exercise or how many did you do? _____

   3. What category of fitness does this activity or exercise fall under? (circle one)

      A. cardiorespiratory   B. muscular strength and endurance   C. flexibility

Kids in Training for a Healthy and Active Lifestyle

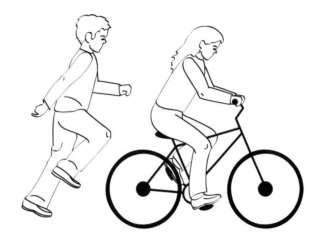

This program is designed to complement the physical education program by getting kids to think about their activity levels. It's simple. If your child chooses to participate in an activity that will further develop physical skills or physical fitness, he or she should fill out the following coupon, have you sign it, and return it to his or her physical education teacher. All returned slips count as extra credit, but the biggest benefit is a stronger and healthier body.

Name _____ **Date** _____

KIDS IN TRAINING FOR A HEALTHY AND ACTIVE LIFESTYLE

Date	Activity	Number of minutes
_____	_____	_____
_____	_____	_____
_____	_____	_____
_____	_____	_____
_____	_____	_____
_____	_____	_____
_____	_____	_____

Parent or guardian signature _____

From *Physical Education Assessment Toolkit* by Liz Giles-Brown, 2006, Champaign, IL: Human Kinetics.

Make Time to Strategize

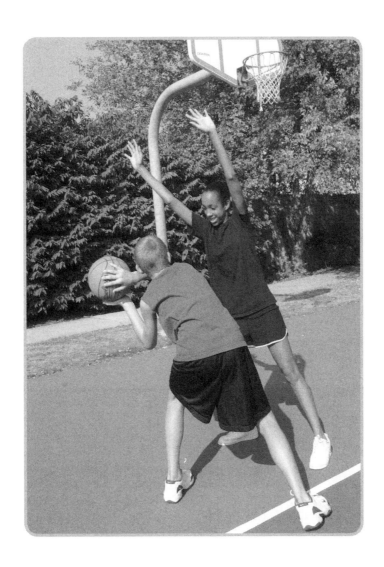

eeing kids think about strategy as they participate in physical activities is rewarding. When they are able to bring strategy into play, they have attained a skill level that allows them to direct their attention outward instead of having to focus on the movement itself. This chapter is dedicated to assessing students' ability to apply strategies to the types of games that children and adults enjoy participating in. All the assessment forms discussed in this chapter are available for reproduction on the accompanying CD-ROM.

The Idea

We all enjoy standing back to observe kids using skills that they have mastered and applying specific strategies as they participate in quality competition. When thinking about teaching and assessing knowledge of and use of strategy, timing is everything. Finding the correct time relies heavily on proper identification of students' skill levels, habits, interactions, and use of virtues. To work on strategy, students must have a solid skill foundation, with most students at least in the practicing stage of skill development. At that level, they can attend to what is going on in their environment instead of having to pay close attention to the skills themselves. Because much strategy work relies on group interaction, students must also have positive interaction habits so that the group members can come to consensus and solve conflicts.

Assessments

The assessments in this section give students opportunities to demonstrate their knowledge and understanding of strategy so that they can more readily apply it to activities. The strategy assessments are broken up into four sections: written assessments, self-assessments, peer or opponent rating assessments, and strategy application. Like most assessment templates in this resource, these templates will fit into any curriculum. Blank spaces allow you to fill in the activities of your choice. Some assessments work well as formative assessments, whereas others work better as summative assessments at the culmination of the unit.

Written Assessments

The chapter contains five written assessment templates. I'm on Offense! (form 7.1) and I'm on Defense! (form 7.2) are simple knowledge assessments that will let you know what strategies students are thinking about applying when they are participating in various types of games. You can use these assessments with any type of game in which strategy can be applied to offense or defense. For example, they could be used in a basketball unit and then in a badminton unit because both activities use the concepts of offense and defense.

Are You Ready? (form 7.3) and What Is Your Intent? (form 7.4) address two strategies—maintaining an athletic ready position and concealing intent—common to many games. Some students understand both concepts; they are always down and ready in almost every situation and they tend not to give away their next move. Other students really need to think about and process these concepts. These two assessments will tell you whether students really understand the strategies in relationship to the activities of the unit.

Strategize! (form 7.5) is more than just a knowledge assessment because it requires students to apply their knowledge of which skills to use in certain situations. Instead of providing the situation and having students choose the best skill, the assessment gives students the skills for the unit and asks them to describe situations in which it would be best to use them. For tips on using these forms, see "Putting It Into Practice: Written Assessments" on page 158.

Self-Assessments

Self-assessment is always a good way to get students to reflect on their performance, but in this situation it serves an additional purpose. Self-assessment provides you with another way to get students to process the information or concepts that you want them to learn. The more and varied ways that you can get kids to process information, the more likely it is that they will retain it for the long haul. The self-assessments seen in Invasion Games—Self-Assessment (form 7.6), Target Games—Self-Assessment (form 7.7), Net Games—Self-Assessment (form 7.8), and Fielding Games—Self-Assessment (form 7.9) can be used quickly and efficiently to reinforce the strategy focus of the lesson or unit. For tips on using these forms, see "Putting It Into Practice: Self-Assessments" on page 159.

Peer or Opponent Rating Assessments

Invasion Games—Peer Assessment (form 7.10), Net Games—Peer Assessment (form 7.11), Fielding Games—Peer Assessment (form 7.12), and Target Games—Peer Assessment (form 7.13) are similar to the self-assessments. But because someone else is doing the rating, more accountability is present. For invasion games and net games, students assess their opponents' use of strategy after they have participated in the activity with them. For target and fielding games, students complete this assessment as a peer assessment, with each person assigned a partner to assess. For tips on using these forms, see "Putting It Into Practice: Peer or Opponent Rating Assessments" on page 159.

Strategy Application Assessments

Many of the activities that children play are invasion games. Getting children of varied skill levels to work cooperatively on applying strategy is not easy. Before you use Offensive Planning (form 7.14) and Defensive Planning (form 7.15), it is best if all students have acquired a skill level that will allow them to focus on strategy. For tips on using these forms, see "Putting It Into Practice: Strategy Application Assessments" on page 160.

Setting Up Everyone for Success

You can do a few things ahead of time to set up students for success when using the strategy assessments in this chapter. The areas to focus on are group size, feedback, objectivity, and practicing virtues.

- When groups are small, more people participate to a larger degree. This statement is true when it comes to just about everything in physical education. Remember this concept when it comes to teaching strategy. Focusing on strategy is easier when done individually, with partners, or with small groups. Large groups need much more time, and students will have difficulty coming to consensus on any one strategy or play. Students may easily get lost in the crowd, whether they want to or not. For instance, students can more easily focus on strategy for net games in a pairs badminton unit than they can in a volleyball unit. In games of invasion, a team of 3 or 4 students can focus on strategy much more easily than a team of 10 can.

- After students have had a few opportunities to use a strategy, you should teach them that if it is not working, they need to look at the feedback available and make changes. They don't necessarily have to abandon a strategy altogether; they may just need to tweak it based on what has been happening. Students need to understand the different types of feedback that they can use to make necessary changes in strategy.

- Learning how to be objective is sometimes difficult for students. Before using the peer-opponent assessments, you should go over the idea of being objective versus letting bias get in the way of good assessment. Students need to learn to separate the performance from the person.

- While students are learning about strategy, you will have many opportunities to focus their attention on the virtues that make classes run smoothly. When strategy is involved, competition is often occurring at some level. Students need to learn that the game is not more important than the people involved. Although quality competition requires each person or team to put forth their best effort to win, it also requires practicing honesty, respect, responsibility, and so on. Drawing students' attention to these virtues and what practicing them will mean for the success of the class will raise consciousness and head off potential problems.

On the pages that follow, you will find lists of ideas for putting each type of assessment form into practice with your students. The lists represent ways in which they have been used before and provide space for you to come up with other ways in which you might use them. Following the "Putting It Into Practice" sections, you will find lesson ideas that target some of the assessments in this chapter. The lessons can be used as written or modified to meet specific needs. The Offensive Planning Lesson Sequence on page 160 represents part of a unit designed to help students further their knowledge and understanding of strategies for invasion games. The target that students are aiming for is to use the strategies for invasion games in order to participate successfully in the game Three Attempts. To implement these steps, students need to have proficient throwing and catching skills and understand the basic strategies for invasion games. This is an application assessment. If students do not have the skills or knowledge, they will not be able to apply them. Finally, you will find all of the forms referred to in this chapter. They are also found on the accompanying CD-ROM for easy printing and use.

Summary

The assessments presented in this chapter on strategy will help students take the skills they have developed to the next level. Remember, however, that you should use these assessments only with classes of students who have developed enough proficiency that they can direct their attention away from direct execution of the skills. Trying to get students to apply offensive strategies in basketball when they haven't yet learned to dribble, pass, or shoot is an exercise in frustration. But getting kids who have the skills to think about how to apply them is extremely rewarding for you and for them. Furthermore, threading the idea of practicing virtues through any unit that involves team or partner strategy will help classes run smoothly and build valuable leadership and team-building skills among students.

PUTTING IT INTO PRACTICE

Written Assessments

- **Process partners**—Partners can work together to complete the assessment and then share ideas with other partnerships or the rest of the class.

- **Homework**—After teaching a series of lessons on strategy for a particular activity, use the assessment as a homework assignment.

- **Watch a game**—If students have opportunities to attend games in the same category (invasion games, net games, and so on), assign them to watch a game (high school or college level), focus on the subject of the assessment, and then complete the assignment.

- **Team assignment**—If you have assigned students to teams for a unit or length of time, part of the team's responsibility could be to complete the assessment by a certain date using consensus decision making.

- **Closure**—During part of the class closure for the unit, students could add to their written assessments as they learn new information so that they complete them at the end of the unit.

- Other ways in which this type of assessment could be used:

_____

_____

_____

Self-Assessments

■ **Prime and assess**—Give students the assessment to look at before they participate in the class activity and tell them that they will be responsible for filling it out at the end of the class period.

■ **Mental notes**—Give students one form at the beginning of the unit and tell them that near the end of the unit you will ask them to complete it as a self-assessment. After each class period ask them to look at the form and put a pencil mark or make a mental note of where they fall on the rating scale. This way students are processing the strategies not only during class but also as a closure before they head out the door.

■ **Comparisons**—Have students complete the self-assessment and then have them participate in the peer or opponent rating assessment described in the next section. Then ask them to compare the two.

■ Other ways in which this type of assessment could be used:

_____

_____

_____

Peer or Opponent Rating Assessments

■ **One at a time**—As students compete against each other, you can direct them to focus on one assessment item at a time. After a given time ask them to stop and rate their opponent on that one item.

■ **Competition shuffle**—For this activity, students place a number in the line for their opponent instead of shading. This method allows more than one person to use the rating sheet. For the first competition students use the number 1. For the second competition they use the number 2, and so on. As students participate in a competitive activity for a specific time interval, have them take along their peer assessment sheets. After the given time or at the end of a game, they trade papers with their opponent and make decisions about where to place the number on each line. This system will show students how they are progressing. At the same time they will be processing the strategies in two different ways before each new challenge.

■ **Looking for progress**—Each time a student participates in an activity with a different opponent, he or she can use this assessment and date it. As students collect each assessment they can compare it to those they did previously and look for improvement or target areas on which they need to focus.

■ Other ways in which this type of assessment could be used:

_____

_____

_____

Strategy Application Assessments

- **Teamwork**—Have students work in small teams in order to complete the assessment and try out their plans.
- **Player–coach**—Individual students, acting as player–coaches, can come up with an offensive or defensive plan as homework and be assigned a day to implement it with their teammates.
- **Co-captains**—Partnerships on a team can come up with an offensive or defensive plan and act as co-captains when it is their turn to introduce it to their other teammates and implement it during class.
- **Sideline work**—Teams rotating out of competition can use that time to work on an offensive or defensive plan and then try it out during their turn for game play. The goal can be to finish by a certain time and implement it by the end of the unit.
- Other ways in which this type of assessment could be used:

_____

_____

_____

Offensive Planning Lesson Sequence

CONCEPT FOCUS

Offensive strategies

SKILL FOCUS

Throwing, catching, and pivoting

EQUIPMENT AND MATERIALS

An Offensive Planning assessment (form 7.14) and a pencil for each team, three small balls that students can successfully throw and catch for each game, boundary markers, one small goal or target for each game, a poster or whiteboard with the following list of strategies on display so that you and students can refer to it:

Offensive Strategy

- I always need to be ready to move, and I should not stand in one area for too long. If I don't move I am easier to guard, and my teammates will have difficulty getting me the ball.
- I can use fakes to conceal my intent.
- I need to move into open spaces to get open for a pass.
- I need to communicate respectfully with my teammates to help the team work more efficiently.

Defensive Strategy

▓ If I'm always in a good athletic ready position, I will increase my success in guarding my opponent.

▓ To play good defense, I need to stay between the goal and the person I am guarding.

▓ I will increase my chances of intercepting the ball if I can always see both the person I am guarding and the ball.

▓ If I lose the person I am guarding, I need to communicate with my teammates that I need someone to help out.

TEACHING AND LEARNING ACTIVITIES

The Game: Three Attempts

▓ **Objective**—The basic version requires students to use throwing and catching skills to invade another team's space to try to score.

▓ **Playing area**—The playing area can be an open space, either outside or inside, marked off with boundary lines. The amount of space given to each team will depend on the amount of space available for small-sided games. To allow for maximum participation, keep teams small, with either three or four players each.

Rules

▓ The team on offense gets three attempts to score, whether successful or not.

▓ If the ball hits the floor or a team scores a point, they begin again until they have made three attempts. A team may score all three times.

▓ After three attempts, the offensive team plays defense and the defensive team switches to offense.

▓ The offensive team begins play with a ball at the end of the playing area. They may move the ball into scoring position by passing to one another but may not run with the ball.

▓ When a player is in possession of the ball, he or she may pivot but may not run or walk with the ball.

▓ Defensive players may guard their opponents in an attempt to intercept a pass or force a bad pass, but they may not grab or hit the ball out of anyone's hands.

▓ You can set up scoring in several ways. To score, players may either hit a target or throw into a goal. No special equipment is needed. Any ball can be used.

▓ Because this game does not use goalkeepers, the targets or goals should be placed outside the playing area, behind a boundary line. No offensive or defensive player may go into that area unless play is stopped and the player is going to retrieve a ball.

▓ All rules for safety apply. No physical contact is allowed, and defensive players must be at least an arm's length away from offensive players. Students may switch players to defend but may not double-team. By practicing the virtues important in quality competition, students can referee their own games.

Step 1: Recognizing a Need

When dealing with strategy, the best approach may be to let the students recognize the need for one. One way to achieve this is to give the directions for the activity and just begin play with no talk of strategy. Often, after a few failed attempts, students will ask if they can have some time to come up with a strategy. This is the perfect opportunity to take a step toward the target, with the best part being that it was the students' idea.

Step 2: Focused Attention

During this step in the process, students get a chance to focus on the strategies that they need to use to increase their success rate.

Directions

1. Taking a cue from the students, direct the class to refer to the strategy lists for this activity. Tell them that they are ready to start focusing on the strategies used in invasion games and that they are going to play the game again but for specific time periods. Each time they finish a period, they will gather and choose a specific area of focus.

2. Start by reading the first offensive and defensive strategy on the list. Tell them that before each attempt at the game, both teams must get together. Members repeat the strategy focus until time is called and they gather with you. If they are playing offense, they repeat the offensive strategy focus. If they are playing defense, they repeat the defensive strategy. This method will help students commit the strategies to memory. If students forget the words, they can look on the poster or whiteboard and read them, but each person must repeat the strategy before the play begins.

3. Repeat this process until students have gone through all the strategies.

Step 3: Player–Coach

This step in the process introduces the player–coach role. This step will give each student a chance to try out his or her ideas about strategy.

Directions

1. Tell students that the items listed on the board are what each person must do to make the team work efficiently but that strategy becomes more specific at times.

2. Ask them to gather with their team and come to consensus on the following question: "How can an offensive strategy be made more specific?" (A strategy becomes more specific when team members do particular jobs to carry out a play or plan.) Ask students to stand in a circle and discuss possible answers. After a minute or two ask groups to volunteer their ideas. Lead them to the correct answer.

3. When students return to play, tell them that each offensive team member will take a turn being the team player–coach for an attempt on offense. The job of the player–coach is to give each player specific directions about what he or she will do to gain an advantage over the defense and score. Each player must understand his or her job before the offense makes an attempt.

4. As teams try the plans or plays, students should be thinking about what makes the plays work or what they might need to change.

5. While the offensive team is working with their player–coach, the defense should review their defensive strategies and assess whether the strategies are working. They can make any changes they wish as long as the team can come to consensus. After both teams have played offense and defense and all students have had a chance to be the player–coach, the students are ready to move on to step 4.

Step 4: Offensive Planning

Based on all the trials, students will have a chance to develop one of their best offensive strategies.

Directions

1. Gather the teams and tell them that they will have a chance to use the experience of all their previous trials to develop one offensive plan for their team.

2. Hand out the assessment (Offensive Planning, form 7.14) and go over the directions. Remind students that as they work to come to consensus on their play, they need to think about the list of offensive strategies on the board. They also need to reflect on their previous trials when they were under the direction of the various player–coaches.

3. As they make decisions about their play, one person from the group should record what they have decided.

4. Students need to make their directions specific so that when read by someone else they can be understood. All team members need to understand what their jobs are in order to carry out the plan.

5. After the teams have come up with their plans, resume play with each team carrying out their play in an attempt to score.

Other ways in which this type of assessment could be used:

_____

_____

_____

I'm on Offense!

Name _____ **Date** _____

Directions: Explain two offensive strategies that you can use to increase your chances of being successful when participating in _____.

1. _____

   _____

   _____

   _____

   _____

2. _____

   _____

   _____

   _____

   _____

Assessment: Your work will be scored according to the criteria in the following rubric. Use this information to self-assess your work before you hand it in.

4	Excellent work! You went above and beyond!	Two specific offensive strategies are provided. Artwork, specific examples, or details that support answers are included.
3	Good work. Everything is here!	Two specific offensive strategies are provided.
2	Good attempt. Just a few things are missing. Would you like to try again?	At least one specific offensive strategy is provided.
1	Let's be sure that you understand. I recommend that you try this one again. See me for more explanation.	The offensive strategies provided are inaccurate or not specific to the sport.

From *Physical Education Assessment Toolkit* by Liz Giles-Brown, 2006, Champaign, IL: Human Kinetics.

I'm on Defense!

Name _____ **Date** _____

Directions: Explain two defensive strategies that you can use to increase your chances of being successful when participating in _____.

1. _____

   _____

   _____

   _____

   _____

   _____

2. _____

   _____

   _____

   _____

   _____

Assessment: Your work will be scored according to the criteria in the following rubric. Use this information to self-assess your work before you hand it in.

4	Excellent work! You went above and beyond!	Two specific defensive strategies are provided. Artwork, specific examples, or details that support answers are included.
3	Good work. Everything is here!	Two specific defensive strategies are provided.
2	Good attempt. Just a few things are missing. Would you like to try again?	At least one specific defensive strategy is provided.
1	Let's be sure that you understand. I recommend that you try this one again. See me for more explanation.	The defensive strategies provided are inaccurate or are not specific to the sport.

From *Physical Education Assessment Toolkit* by Liz Giles-Brown, 2006, Champaign, IL: Human Kinetics.

FORM 7.3 **Are You Ready?**

Name _____ **Date** _____

Directions: We are involved in a _____ unit. Maintaining a good athletic ready position is important in all physical activities. This position gives players an advantage when competing in all types of games. In the spaces provided explain what a good athletic ready position looks like and list two specific advantages that it offers a person who maintains it when participating in _____.

_____

_____

_____

_____

_____

_____

_____

_____

_____

Assessment: Your work will be scored according to the criteria in the following rubric. Use this information to self-assess your work before you hand it in.

4	Excellent work! You went above and beyond!	A complete, accurate description of an athletic ready position and two correct and specific advantages of maintaining a good athletic ready position are provided. Artwork, specific examples, or details that support answers are included.
3	Good work. Everything is here!	A complete, accurate description of an athletic ready position and two correct and specific advantages of maintaining a good athletic ready position are provided.
2	Good attempt. Just a few things are missing. Would you like to try again?	Most of the response is complete and correct. The description of an athletic ready position may be lacking minor details, or an advantage identified may be incorrect or incomplete.
1	Let's be sure that you understand. I recommend that you try this one again. See me for more explanation.	Little of the response is correct or complete. The description of an athletic ready position and the advantages listed are either missing, incorrect, or incomplete.

From *Physical Education Assessment Toolkit* by Liz Giles-Brown, 2006, Champaign, IL: Human Kinetics.

What Is Your Intent?

Name _____ **Date** _____

Directions: Jason was watching Julie play _____. He noticed that he was never quite sure what she was going to do next when she was on offense. He really wanted to know how she did such a good job of fooling her opponent. List three things that you think Julie might be doing to avoid revealing her intent when she is on offense.

1. _____

   _____

   _____

   _____

   _____

2. _____

   _____

   _____

   _____

   _____

3. _____

   _____

   _____

   _____

   _____

Assessment: Your work will be scored according to the criteria in the following rubric. Use this information to self-assess your work before you hand it in.

4	Excellent work! You went above and beyond!	Three correct, complete, specific ways in which Julie could conceal her intent are provided. Artwork, specific examples, or details that support answers are included.
3	Good work. Everything is here!	Three correct, complete, specific ways in which Julie could conceal her intent are provided.
2	Good attempt. Just a few things are missing. Would you like to try again?	At least two correct, complete, specific ways in which Julie could conceal her intent are provided.
1	Let's be sure that you understand. I recommend that you try this one again. See me for more explanation.	Fewer than two correct, complete, specific ways in which Julie could conceal her intent are provided.

From *Physical Education Assessment Toolkit* by Liz Giles-Brown, 2006, Champaign, IL: Human Kinetics.

Strategize!

Name _____ **Date** _____

Describe a situation in which using each of the skills listed would be the best strategy.

1. _____   -   _____

_____

_____

2. _____   -   _____

_____

_____

3. _____   -   _____

_____

_____

4. _____   -   _____

_____

Assessment: Your work will be scored according to the criteria in the following rubric. Use this information to self-assess your work before you hand it in.

4	Excellent work! You went above and beyond!	For each skill listed, a specific description of a game situation in which the skill would be the best strategy to use is provided. Artwork, specific examples, or details that support answers are included.
3	Good work. Everything is here!	For each skill listed, a specific description of a game situation in which the skill would be the best strategy to use is provided.
2	Good attempt. Just a few things are missing. Would you like to try again?	For three skills listed, specific descriptions of game situations in which those skills would be the best strategy to use are provided.
1	Let's be sure that you understand. I recommend that you try this one again. See me for more explanation.	For one or two skills listed, specific descriptions of game situations in which those skills would be the best strategy to use are provided.

From *Physical Education Assessment Toolkit* by Liz Giles-Brown, 2006, Champaign, IL: Human Kinetics.

Invasion Games—Self-Assessment

Name _____ **Date** _____

Directions: Assess yourself by shading in the learning line following each strategy that you use during _____.

1. I consistently move to the open spaces to get open when I'm playing offense.

never	some of the time	most of the time

2. I'm always ready and maintain a good athletic position. My opponent has a hard time guarding me when I'm playing offense.

never	some of the time	a lot of the time	most of the time

3. I make it hard for my opponent to get open, pass, or score when I'm playing defense.

never	some of the time	most of the time

4. I communicate well with my teammates so that we all work more efficiently as a group. I am open-minded and willing to listen to feedback from teammates.

never	some of the time	most of the time

From *Physical Education Assessment Toolkit* by Liz Giles-Brown, 2006, Champaign, IL: Human Kinetics.

Target Games—Self-Assessment

Name _____ **Date** _____

Directions: Assess yourself by shading in the learning line following each strategy that you use during _____.

1. I am relaxed and able to stay focused on each attempt.

never	some of the time	most of the time

2. I do not rush through a shot. I take my time and concentrate on using my best skills.

never	some of the time	most of the time

3. I do not get upset with myself when I make a mistake. I assess the performance and attempt to make adjustments on the next trial.

never	some of the time	most of the time

From *Physical Education Assessment Toolkit* by Liz Giles-Brown, 2006, Champaign, IL: Human Kinetics.

Net Games—Self-Assessment

Name _____ **Date** _____

Directions: Assess yourself by shading in the learning line following each strategy that you use during _____.

1. I maintain an athletic ready position and am focused on the play. It is difficult for my opponent to score.

never   some of the time   most of the time

| |
| |

2. I attempt to send the ball or object to open areas so that my opponent has to move to play it.

never   some of the time   most of the time

| |
| |

3. I use a variety of shots so that it is hard for my opponent to predict what I will do from one play to the next.

never   some of the time   most of the time

| |
| |

Fielding Games—Self-Assessment

Name _____ **Date** _____

Directions: Assess yourself by shading in the learning line following each strategy that you use during _____.

1. I try to send the ball or object to the open spaces so that fielders have to move to stop it when I'm playing offense.

never   some of the time   most of the time

| |
| |

2. I maintain an athletic ready position and stay focused on the ball. I am never caught standing up or not paying attention when I'm playing defense.

never   some of the time   most of the time

| |
| |

3. I move to get in front of the ball or object when it is hit to my area when I'm playing defense.

never   some of the time   most of the time

| |
| |

4. I am ready and move to back up teammates when necessary when I'm playing defense.

never   some of the time   most of the time

| |
| |

Invasion Games—Peer Assessment

Performer's Name _____ **Assessor's Name** _____

Directions: Assess your classmate or opponent by shading in the learning line followi_ng each strategy that he or she uses during team activities.

1. My opponent consistently moves to the open spaces and gets open when playing offense.

never	some of the time	most of the time

2. My opponent is always ready on offense. He or she maintains a good athletic ready position and is difficult to guard.

never	some of the time	most of the time

3. My opponent defends me well, making it hard for me to get open, pass, or score.

never	some of the time	most of the time

4. My opponent communicates well with his or her teammates so that they work more efficiently as a group.

never	some of the time	most of the time

Net Games—Peer Assessment

Performer's Name _____ **Assessor's Name** _____

Directions: Assess your opponent by shading in the learning line following each strategy that he or she uses during net activities.

1. My opponent maintains an athletic ready position and is focused on the play. It is difficult for me to score.

never	some of the time	most of the time

2. My opponent attempts to send the ball or object to the open areas so that I have to move to play it.

never	some of the time	most of the time

3. My opponent uses a variety of shots so that it is hard for me to predict what he or she is going to do from one play to the next.

never	some of the time	most of the time

4. My opponent covers space efficiently by consistently being in the position that gives him or her the best coverage.

never	some of the time	most of the time

Fielding Games—Peer Assessment

Performer's Name _____ **Assessor's Name** _____

Directions: Assess your partner by shading in the learning line following each strategy that he or she uses during fielding games.

    1. My partner sends the ball or object to the open spaces so that fielders have to move to stop it.

never	some of the time	most of the time

    2. My partner always maintains an athletic ready position.

never	some of the time	most of the time

    3. My partner moves to get in front of the ball or object when it is hit to his or her area.

never	some of the time	most of the time

    4. My partner moves to back up teammates when necessary.

never	some of the time	most of the time

From *Physical Education Assessment Toolkit* by Liz Giles-Brown, 2006, Champaign, IL: Human Kinetics.

FORM 7.13 **Target Games—Peer Assessment**

Performer's Name _____ **Assessor's Name** _____

Directions: Assess your opponent or partner by shading in the learning line following each strategy that he or she uses during target activities.

    1. My partner is relaxed and able to stay focused on each attempt.

never	some of the time	most of the time

    2. My partner does not rush through a shot. He or she takes time to concentrate on using his or her skills.

never	some of the time	most of the time

    3. My partner does not get upset with himself or herself after making a mistake. He or she assesses the performance and attempts to make adjustments on the next trial.

never	some of the time	most of the time

From *Physical Education Assessment Toolkit* by Liz Giles-Brown, 2006, Champaign, IL: Human Kinetics.

Offensive Planning

Name _____ **Date** _____

Directions: Planning offensive strategy can give your team an advantage. Using what you know and understand about offensive strategies in _____, come to consensus on an offensive plan that you can use to gain an advantage over the opposing team. Using diagrams and symbols, write a brief description of your plan and then put your plan into action. Be sure to include what players should do to restart the plan if it does not result in a goal or score.

Assessment: Your work will be scored according to the criteria in the following rubric. Use this information to self-assess your work before you hand it in.

4	Excellent work! You went above and beyond!	The plan clearly shows how the offense will gain an advantage over the opposing team. It is a clear application of offensive strategy. The plan is diagrammed with symbols that make it clear what every team member is supposed to do. The description of the plan is complete, detailed, and easy to understand. In addition, directions describe what team members should do to restart the plan if it doesn't result in a goal.
3	Good work. Everything is here!	The plan clearly shows how the offense will gain an advantage over the opposing team. It is a clear application of offensive strategy. The plan is diagrammed with symbols that make it clear what every team member is supposed to do. The description of the plan is complete and easy to understand.
2	Good attempt. Just a few things are missing. Would you like to try this one again?	The plan is not completely clear in showing how the offense will gain an advantage over the opposing team. It is not a clear application of offensive strategy. The plan is missing some symbols that might make it easier to understand. The description is incomplete and is difficult to understand in places.
1	Let's be sure that you understand. I recommend that you try this one again. See me for more explanation.	The plan does not show how the offense will gain an advantage over the opposing team. It is not an application of offensive strategy. The plan is missing many symbols that would make it easier to understand. The description contains little detail and is difficult to follow.

From *Physical Education Assessment Toolkit* by Liz Giles-Brown, 2006, Champaign, IL: Human Kinetics.

Defensive Planning

Name _____ **Date** _____

Directions: Planning defensive strategy can give your team an advantage and quickly move you from a defensive position to an offensive position. Using what you know and understand about defensive strategies in _____, come to consensus on a defensive strategy that you can use to gain an advantage over the opposing team and quickly make the transition to offense. Using diagrams and symbols, write a brief description of your plan and be ready to put it into action.

Assessment: Your work will be scored according to the criteria in the following rubric. Use this information to self-assess your work before you hand it in.

4	Excellent work! You went above and beyond!	The plan clearly shows how the defense will gain an advantage over the opposing team. It is a clear application of defensive strategy. The plan is diagrammed with symbols that make it clear what every team member is supposed to do. The description of the plan is complete, detailed, and easy to understand. Additional details are included to aid understanding.
3	Good work. Everything is here!	The plan clearly shows how the defense will gain an advantage over the opposing team. It is a clear application of defensive strategy. The plan is diagrammed with symbols that make it clear what every team member is supposed to do. The description of the plan is complete and easy to understand.
2	Good attempt. Just a few things are missing. Would you like to try this one again?	The plan is not completely clear in showing how the defense will gain an advantage over the opposing team. It is not a clear application of defensive strategy. The plan is missing some symbols that might make it easier to understand. The description is incomplete and is difficult to understand in places.
1	Let's be sure that you understand. I recommend that you try this one again. See me for more explanation.	The plan does not show how the defense will gain an advantage over the opposing team. It is not an application of defensive strategy. The plan is missing many symbols that would make it easier to understand. The description contains little detail and is difficult to follow.

8

CHAPTER

Decorate With Content

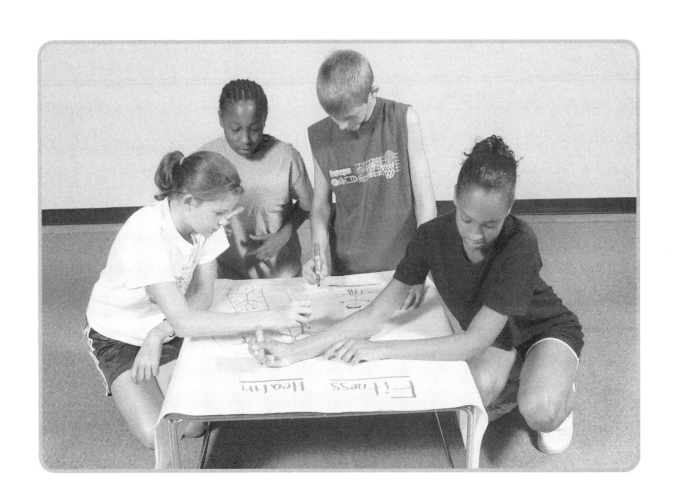

This chapter deals with decorating the physical education teaching space with content that can foster learning and support assessment. Displaying posters that complement the curriculum and that you incorporate into lessons helps students make more connections.

The Idea

The idea is a simple one. Content posters will not only reinforce the skills and concepts that you are teaching but also create a way in which you can quickly and efficiently do formative assessment. Nine posters are included on the accompanying CD-ROM. These posters can be printed at a large size (up to 25.5 inches by 33 inches) or on a regular desktop printer (8.5 inches by 11 inches), and they can be printed in full color or in black and white. You can use the posters with the units or lesson ideas provided in the book or with a new unit that you develop. When placed on the walls of the teaching space, they provide a point of reference useful throughout the learning process. The posters also provide students who are strong visual learners another way to focus on the material being taught.

The Posters

All the posters in this section support learning in physical education. More specifically, they support the assessments presented in this resource. Is It All About the Skills? (poster 8.1) draws attention to all the things besides physical skills that go into a quality physical education experience. You can use Stop, Think, and Make Changes (poster 8.2) as an informal reflection tool. These posters complement the assessments found in chapters 2 and 3.

Skill Stages—Where Am I? (poster 8.3) will get students to think about the stages that they go through when learning skills. From there, they can begin focusing on what they need to do to move forward in their skill development.

What Type of Feedback Will You Use to Improve Your Skills and Performance? (poster 8.4) is a helpful reference when teaching students how to give peer feedback and how to become self-directed learners by using feedback resulting from movement. Both posters are helpful in supporting motor skill development and the assessments in chapter 4.

How Can I Use Space? (poster 8.5) helps illustrate movement concepts that students need to

be thinking about when participating in a wide variety of activities. Laws to Move By (poster 8.6) provides you with a way to refer to the concepts that support various skills. When teaching a lesson, you will find having a reference point useful in helping students understand how they can use their knowledge and understanding of concepts to improve performance. You can use these two posters in conjunction with the assessments found in chapter 5.

Thinking About Health-Related Fitness (poster 8.7) and Thinking About Skill-Related Fitness (poster 8.8) are good examples of how to thread health- and skill-related fitness into lessons in which fitness may not be the primary focus. These posters can help students make connections between the physical activities that they do and their health- and skill-related fitness development. Making these connections regularly instead of once or twice a year during a unit focused on fitness will help make them part of students' everyday thinking. These posters can effectively support the learning and assessments in chapter 6.

Make Time to Strategize (poster 8.9) is useful when students have moved forward in their skill development and are ready to start thinking about strategy. The assessments in chapter 7 focus on offensive and defensive strategies used in different types of games. You can use this poster as a way to refer to the strategies that you are focusing on during a unit.

Setting Up Everyone for Success

Many students are strong visual learners. Being able to see and read what you are talking about will help those students learn the material more completely. Some students have a difficult time reading. Take time to go over the posters, point to the words, and make sure that all students know what they say. Use a laser pointer to point to each word so that students know where to look.

On the pages that follow, you will find a list of ideas for putting the posters into practice with your students. The list represents ways in which it has been used before and provides space for you to come up with other ways in which you might use it. Following the "Putting It Into Practice" section, you will find lesson ideas that target some of the assessments in this chapter. The lesson can be used as written or modified to meet specific needs. The Content Posters Lesson Activity on page 178 can be used as a closure activity in a series of lessons at the beginning of the school year or just after you display the posters. The activity is part of a lesson, not a lesson itself. This activity will familiarize students with the content of each poster so that they can begin to make connections between what is represented on the posters and the physical education lessons. You will find the posters referred to in this chapter on the accompanying CD-ROM for easy printing and use.

Summary

The posters presented in this chapter can have a profound effect on what students remember from day to day. The simple act of decorating the teaching space with the concepts you want students to learn and use on a daily basis is another way to help them learn. In addition, it provides another way in which you can check for understanding and do quick formative assessments.

PUTTING IT INTO PRACTICE

Content Posters

You can use content posters in several ways to support student learning in physical education: as part of the assessment for a unit, as a reference point during a lesson to support the learning, as part of class closure, or on other occasions.

- **Off the cuff**—When teaching a lesson, you may come across an opportunity to use a content poster to illustrate a point or make a connection that will support learning. Posters on the walls are an excellent teaching aid.

- **Threads**—When planning a unit, you choose the focus from many possibilities. For instance, during the badminton unit in chapter 11 the concept focus is strategy. But you could make connections to other concepts during this unit. During a unit students may need to think about force production, health-related fitness components, or skill-related fitness components. Content posters can get students to think about the threads that bind together everything they do in physical education. Revisiting concepts focused on in previous units of instruction helps students remember and make applications. The content posters serve this purpose because they include information that supports learning and helps you and your students make more connections.

- **Process partners**—This resource often uses the idea of assigning processing partners. Chapter 9 explains this idea fully, and chapters 10, 11, and 12 use it extensively. You can use the content posters with partners by drawing students' attention to a particular poster and asking them to come to consensus on answers to a question.

- **Prime and question**—As students walk in the door for physical education class, draw their attention to a specific poster. Tell them that at the end of the class period you will ask them a question based on what they do during the class period and that poster. Ask them to be thinking of the connection between the two as the class progresses. At the end of class ask them a specific question. By priming them at the beginning of class, you increase the likelihood of getting higher quality answers.

(continued)

(continued)

- **Quick check**—Having a box of scrap paper and a container of pencils enables you to use the posters as an assessment tool. Ask students to write answers to specific questions, using the posters as a reference point. For instance, you could ask students to look at the poster Thinking About Health-Related Fitness (poster 8.7) and answer the following question: "Think about physical education class and write down one cardiorespiratory activity that we did when your heart and lungs were thanking you." Have them write the answer, put their name on the paper, and hand it to you. After all the papers are in, ask students to share what they wrote. This method provides a quick check to see whether students really understand the different types of health-related fitness activities.
- **Partner questions**—Instruct one partner to use the poster that the class is focusing on to design a question to ask his or her partner. Then have them switch roles.
- **Find the poster**—Instruct partnerships, groups, or teams to read the content posters that are on the wall and choose one that complements or supports the learning that took place during the class period. Gather them back together and ask them to share their ideas.
- Other ways in which this type of assessment could be used:

_____

_____

_____

Content Posters Lesson Activity

CONCEPT FOCUS

All physical education concepts represented on the posters

SKILL FOCUS

Reading, listening skills, making connections between the lessons and concepts on posters

EQUIPMENT AND MATERIALS

CD player, quiet slow music with no words (cool-down music), posters, any equipment necessary for the rest of the lesson

TEACHING AND LEARNING ACTIVITIES

- **Setup**—Display the posters around the room so that students can move around and read them.
- **Poster connections**—By participating in this activity, students will begin thinking about the connections that they can make between the physical education lesson and the concepts that support or contribute to successful participation and learning.

Directions

1. When appropriate (as a cool-down or closure activity) tell students that when the music starts they should walk around the room and look at the words and pictures on the posters. Tell them that as they walk around they should think about how the posters connect in some way to the lesson or activity that they just participated in.

2. After a minute or two, stop the music. Tell them that on the signal to move, they should stand in front of the poster that they feel has a clear connection to the lesson or activity. This activity should take less than a minute.

3. When all students have chosen a poster, instruct them to form a circle with the other students at the same poster. They then go around the circle and share the connections that they made.

Note: By doing this activity during several lessons, students become familiar with the posters and more aware of the threads that bind together what they do.

Clipboard Closure and Processing Partners

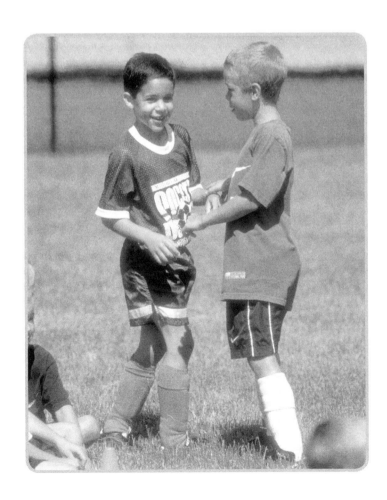

Formal class closure is not a new idea, but failing to include it can easily occur in the rush of finishing one class and beginning another. Closing the class by having students focus on the main concepts or ideas leaves them with the important stuff on their minds. In an attempt to get as much activity into a class period, teachers sometimes end the activity and send students off without helping them refocus on the content of the lesson. On other occasions, teachers have students gather in one area and ask them a question that only a few students get a chance to answer. This chapter is dedicated to exploring an engaging, time-efficient way of closing class. All the open-ended statement lists discussed in this chapter are available for reproduction on the accompanying CD-ROM.

The Idea

Clipboard closure statements used with processing partners is a way in which students can refocus on the content, share ideas with at least one other person, practice respectful listening skills, and be held accountable for engaging in the process. This method is not a formal assessment, but it is useful in assessing whether students are gaining an understanding of the lesson content.

Clipboard Closure Statements

We all use questions during lessons to get kids to think deeper, to see what they remember, or to be sure that they understand what we are trying to teach them. One questioning technique that successfully engages all students is using strategically placed, open-ended statements as an informal method of formative assessment. Instead of asking questions with one correct answer, we can ask students to complete statements that have many correct answers and often enable every student to answer successfully at some level of thinking.

The forms in this chapter provide lists of open-ended statements that you can use for this purpose. You can print them out and place them on the clipboard for easy access at the end of each class period. If you're following the backward planning method of unit development, you can choose the closure statements to complement the assessments targeted for the unit. The process of

identifying these questions before beginning will help you see the target more clearly, which means that you will be able to help students see it more clearly too.

Processing Partners

When we ask questions of a group in physical education classes, we often have time to take only one or two answers. If we called on every student every time we asked a question, we would use up the entire class period. At other times, the same few students raise their hands to answer every question. A student could easily go an entire year without attempting or being required to answer a single question. Processing partners involves spending some time at the beginning of the unit to set up the system, but after students become familiar with it, the system saves time and promotes learning. At the beginning of the unit, you assign students to a processing partner; partners will stand and face each other during the closure of each class period. At this point you present the open-ended statement for the day, and partnerships come to consensus on an answer. When they have reached consensus they sit down to signal that they are finished. This procedure lets you know which students have completed the task and are ready to share their answers.

With this system, all students have the opportunity to answer and be heard for each closure statement posed, even though you may not call on them to share with the entire class. If you set up partners at the beginning of the unit so that students know that they will be working with the same person during each closure, you will reduce transition time. You can change partners after each unit, quarter, or trimester so that students get used to working with different people.

Although this section is dedicated to using the open-ended statements during closure, you can use the procedure quickly and efficiently at any time during a lesson. You can stop the action at any time and ask students to find their processing partners. The transition should take no more than 5 or 10 seconds. When using this strategy during a lesson in which students have been working in an activity or on a specific skill, they can signal that they are finished and ready to share their answer by returning to work again. When two students facing each other must come to consensus on how to finish a statement, each is more likely to be an active participant in the process.

Assessments

The closure statement assessments address the following categories:

- Interactions (form 9.1)
- Virtues (form 9.2)
- Basic Movement Concepts (form 9.3)
- Laws to Move By (form 9.4)
- Flexibility (form 9.5)
- Muscular Strength and Endurance (form 9.6)
- Body Composition (form 9.7)
- Cardiorespiratory Fitness (form 9.8)
- Health-Related Fitness—Principles of Training (form 9.9)
- Skill-Related Fitness (form 9.10)
- Strategy—All Types of Games (form 9.11)
- Strategy—Tag Games (form 9.12)
- Strategy—Net Games (form 9.13)
- Strategy—Target Games (form 9.14)
- Strategy—Invasion Games (form 9.15)
- Strategy—Fielding Games (form 9.16)

You can print all the forms and keep them on a clipboard, ready to use, or you can choose ahead of time which statements to include in each lesson based on the focus of the unit. For example, in the units found in chapters 10, 11, and 12 you can see that the statements chosen for each unit were clearly based on the unit objectives. The statements were chosen to leave students thinking about either the skill focus or the concept focus of each lesson. And because there was more than one focus, the statements came from different categories. Using these open-ended statements at the end of a lesson with a single processing partner is only one option. You can use these statements in many different ways throughout the course of a unit. For tips on using these forms, see "Putting It Into Practice: Clipboard Closure Statements" on page 184.

Setting Up Everyone for Success

When using this teaching and assessment strategy, you can do several things to set up students for success. The first is to make time for students to practice respectful listening and consensus decision making. A section in chapter 1 outlines how to build this activity into a lesson. Practicing these skills will help students not only during this process but also in many other partner and group situations that occur in and out of the school setting. The second way in which you can set up students for success during this process is to post the closure question on a whiteboard and draw attention to it at the beginning of class. For example, as students walk into the gymnasium instruct them to read the whiteboard and be thinking throughout the lesson about how they might complete the statement. This priming will make them conscious of the lesson focus so that they will be thinking about it as the lesson progresses.

On the pages that follow, you will find a list of ideas for putting the assessment forms into practice with your students. The list represents ways in which it has been used before and provides space for you to come up with other ways in which you might use it. Following the "Putting It Into Practice" section, you will find lesson ideas that target some of the assessments in this chapter. The lessons can be used as written or modified to meet specific needs. The Processing Partners Lesson Activity on page 184 can be used to introduce students to the process of using partners and open-ended statements, either during a lesson or as part of the lesson closure. If you are planning to implement this teaching strategy, use this activity at the beginning of the year so that students become familiar with the process and will be able to participate quickly and efficiently. Refer to the units in chapters 10 through 12 to see how this strategy is incorporated into lessons and units. Finally, you will find all of the forms referred to in this chapter. They are also found on the accompanying CD-ROM for easy printing and use.

Summary

The open-ended statements presented in this chapter for processing information during and at the close of class have one major objective: to get all kids thinking about and processing the information that we present in a more active and engaging way. Using processing partners within the lesson gives all students a chance to be heard by someone and holds them more accountable. Closing class by having students focus on the big ideas or concepts of the lesson leaves them thinking about the important stuff. This chapter is about paying more attention to the way that we get students to think about the content of the lesson.

Clipboard Closure Statements

- **Write it down**—Have processing partners write their answers to the statement on a piece of paper and hand it in on the way out of class to increase accountability.

- **Checkout**—Copy the closure statements chosen for the unit onto the unit checkout sheet and have students choose one to answer at the end of each class.

- **Teams**—Ask working teams of students to brainstorm answers that complete the statement, with one person from the team acting as a recorder.

- **Exit answers**—After giving the statement, stand at the door as students leave and have partnerships give their answer on the way out. (Have the line of students waiting to exit stand a distance away from you as you receive answers so that students cannot just repeat the answers that they hear from those ahead of them.)

- **Share**—After two students have come to consensus about how to answer the question, ask them to pair up with another partnership and share their answers.

- Other ways in which this type of assessment could be used:

_____

_____

_____

Processing Partners Lesson Activity

CONCEPT FOCUS

Communication

SKILL FOCUS

Listening skills

EQUIPMENT AND MATERIALS

CD player, upbeat music

TEACHING AND LEARNING ACTIVITIES

- **Setup**—You will need an open space for this activity. No equipment is required.

- **Processing partners**—By participating in this activity, students will not only learn how to participate in processing partners but also review good communication skills. After this initial introductory activity you won't have to do it again when you change partners for the next period (unit, quarter, trimester). You will simply assign new processing partners because students will be familiar with the process.

Directions

1. As students walk into the gym ask them to find an open space. Tell them that they are going to participate in an activity that will teach them how to perform a process called processing partners. Let them know that they will use this process all year to learn and remember more.

2. Tell students that when the music starts they need to move into open spaces and that every time the music stops they need to find someone close to them and stand facing each other. If the class has an odd number of students, each round will have one group of three. Tell students that each time the music stops they need to be standing with someone new.

   Note: Give a quick reminder about being caring and using kind body language when partnering up.

3. Start and stop the music several times. After a few rounds, look to be sure that partners are going to work well together for this first assignment of processing partners. Stop the activity when you are happy with the partnerships. You will use these processing partners for the period that you have designated (unit, quarter, trimester).

4. When you stop the activity, tell students to look closely at their partners because that person will be their processing partner for the period that you have chosen. Tell them that as processing partners, they have the job of processing information to come up with the best possible answers. They may do that during a lesson or at the end of a lesson, but for now they are just going to practice communicating with each other.

5. As students stand facing each other, tell them that you will be giving them some sentences to complete. They need to remain standing until they can come to consensus on the best answer. When they have done that, they sit down to signal that they are finished. Tell them that they must use their time efficiently because they will have only a few minutes to complete each one. If they sit down both partners must know the answer that they agreed on. If they're sitting you may call on them at any time to share their answer. Tell them not to sit down if they are not able to come to consensus on an answer.

6. After each statement, watch students and call time when you feel that they have had long enough or when a good percentage of the class is seated. Call on students to share their answers with the rest of the class. Do not call on students who remain standing.

   Note: If you notice a group that never sits down, work with them to discover the reason.

7. After you have used the statements that you selected, teach the rest of your planned lesson. During class closure, use these partners again and have them complete a statement related to the content of the lesson. Remind students that any time you ask them to stand with their processing partners, they will work with the person to whom they were assigned during this activity.

Activity Statements

Use these ideas to get started. You can develop your own statements tailored to the needs of your students.

- "One way that my partner will know I'm really listening to him or her is . . ."
- "My partner might think that I'm not interested in his or her ideas if . . ."
- "A good processing partner will . . ."
- "If we both feel strongly that our own answer is correct and neither of us is willing to budge we should . . ."
- "The consensus decision-making process is . . ."
- "I can disagree respectfully by . . ."

185

Interactions

Rules are important because without them . . .

Many activities have rules so . . .

When people choose not to follow class rules . . .

When people choose not to follow rules for a specific activity . . .

A conflict is . . .

We can resolve conflicts respectfully by . . .

Good communication sounds like . . .

Good communication can help me be more successful in physical education because . . .

Making good decisions involves . . .

I can show respect for individual differences by . . .

Quality competition is . . .

Two ways in which negative peer pressure could influence me during physical activities are . . .

Two ways in which positive peer pressure could influence me during physical activities are . . .

The first step in solving a problem is . . .

Other open-ended closure statements that can be used to assess students' knowledge and understanding of interactions:

_____

_____

_____

_____

_____

_____

_____

_____

_____

_____

_____

_____

_____

_____

_____

_____

_____

From *Physical Education Assessment Toolkit* by Liz Giles-Brown, 2006, Champaign, IL: Human Kinetics.

FORM 9.2 **Virtues**

Two virtues that I can practice during physical education are . . .

Respect is . . .

Respectfulness looks like . . .

Respectfulness sounds like . . .

Practicing respect in physical education classes is important when . . .

Responsibility is . . .

Responsibility looks like . . .

Responsibility sounds like . . .

Practicing responsibility in physical education classes is important when . . .

Perseverance is . . .

Perseverance looks like . . .

Perseverance sounds like . . .

Practicing perseverance in physical education classes is important when . . .

Self-discipline is . . .

Self-discipline looks like . . .

Self-discipline sounds like . . .

Practicing self-discipline in physical education classes is important when . . .

Honesty is . . .

Honesty looks like . . .

Honesty sounds like . . .

Practicing honesty in physical education classes is important when . . .

Compassion is . . .

(continued)

From *Physical Education Assessment Toolkit* by Liz Giles-Brown, 2006, Champaign, IL: Human Kinetics.

Compassion looks like . . .

Compassion sounds like . . .

Practicing compassion in physical education classes is important when . . .

Courage is . . .

Courage looks like . . .

Courage sounds like . . .

Practicing courage in physical education classes is important when . . .

Trustworthiness is . . .

Trustworthiness looks like . . .

Trustworthiness sounds like . . .

Practicing trustworthiness in physical education classes is important when . . .

Two virtues that a person can work on in physical education are . . .

Practicing virtues can help us reach group goals because . . .

Other open-ended closure statements that can be used to assess students' knowledge and understanding of virtues:

_____

_____

_____

_____

_____

_____

_____

_____

_____

_____

_____

From *Physical Education Assessment Toolkit* by Liz Giles-Brown, 2006, Champaign, IL: Human Kinetics.

Basic Movement Concepts

My body surfaces are . . .

My body can . . .

The shapes that I can make with my body are . . .

Locomotor movements are . . .

Examples of locomotor movements are . . .

Being able to perform lots of different locomotor movements efficiently will help me be more successful when I . . .

Being able to (name of locomotor movement) well is important if I want to be successful when I . . .

Nonlocomotor movements are . . .

Examples of nonlocomotor movements are . . .

Being able to perform many different nonlocomotor movements efficiently will help me be more successful in . . .

Being able to (name of nonlocomotor movement) well is important for successful participation in . . .

Manipulative movements are . . .

Examples of manipulative movements are . . .

Being able to (name of manipulative movement) well is important for successful participation in . . .

The different qualities of movement are . . .

Qualities of time can be . . .

Qualities of force can be . . .

Qualities of flow can be . . .

The pathways my body can move in are . . .

Being able to use changes in pathway is important when I . . .

When I'm _____, if I always move in straight pathways I will . . .

The directions that my body can move in are . . .

Being able to change directions quickly is important in . . .

The levels that my body can move in are . . .

Being able to move quickly using changes of speed, direction, and pathway is an important skill to have to be successful in . . .

Being able to move efficiently at different levels is an important skill to have to be successful in . . .

Other open-ended closure statements that can be used to assess students' knowledge and understanding of basic movement concepts:

_____

_____

_____

From *Physical Education Assessment Toolkit* by Liz Giles-Brown, 2006, Champaign, IL: Human Kinetics.

FORM 9.4 **Laws to Move By**

Science underlies all movement. By learning some of the science that governs movement I can . . .

Internal force production depends on . . .

External factors that affect the force that the body can produce are . . .

Two things that I can change to control the amount of force that I am able to produce with my body are . . .

Two physical skills in which it is necessary to be able to produce the most force possible are . . .

Two physical skills in which it is necessary to be able to adjust and control the amount of force produced are . . .

Two activities that require participants to produce a great amount of force and concentrate on accuracy at the same time are . . .

Levers are . . .

Body levers are made up of . . .

Two physical activities in which levers are used are . . .

Follow-through is . . .

Following through is important when I (name a motor skill) because . . .

A projectile is . . .

Trajectory means . . .

Two things that can affect the trajectory of an object are . . .

A collision is . . .

Two activities in which collisions occur are . . .

The result of a collision depends on . . .

Rebound is . . .

Two activities in which rebounds occur are . . .

Spin is created when . . .

Two types of spin are . . .

A spinning object will always rebound in the direction of the . . .

When topspin is applied an object will . . .

I can apply topspin when I'm (name of motor skill) by . . .

When backspin is applied an object will . . .

I can apply backspin when I'm (name of motor skill) by . . .

Two activities in which I can use spin to gain an advantage are . . .

The angle of rebound depends on . . .

To lessen rebound and increase control, I can . . .

(continued)

Velocity is . . .

Acceleration is . . .

I can increase acceleration by . . .

Speed is . . .

I can increase my speed by . . .

My base of support consists of . . .

Gravity is . . .

My center of gravity is . . .

Stability is . . .

Equilibrium is . . .

Balance is . . .

As my center of gravity moves toward my base of support, I . . .

Stability depends on . . .

Lowering my center of gravity and widening my base of support will . . .

If I want to move quickly I need to raise my center of gravity and move it toward the edge of my . . .

If I wanted to maximize my stability I need to . . .

Balance is important for . . .

Other open-ended closure statements that can be used to assess students' knowledge and understanding of the laws they move by:

_____

_____

_____

_____

_____

_____

_____

_____

_____

_____

_____

_____

From *Physical Education Assessment Toolkit* by Liz Giles-Brown, 2006, Champaign, IL: Human Kinetics.

FORM 9.5 **Flexibility**

Flexibility is the ability to . . .

I'll know that I have high levels of flexibility when . . .

I should try to do flexibility exercises at least . . .

When I do flexibility exercises it should feel . . .

If I do flexibility exercises regularly my muscles will become . . .

If I have poor flexibility my muscles have become . . .

Two health benefits of maintaining healthy levels of flexibility are . . .

I will know that my flexibility is improving when . . .

When I perform static stretches I should . . .

Highly flexible people are less likely to hurt themselves when they . . .

Stretching shouldn't . . .

Static stretches are . . .

Three activities that require healthful levels of flexibility to be successful are . . .

Other open-ended closure statements that can be used to assess students' knowledge and understanding of flexibility:

_____

_____

_____

_____

_____

_____

_____

_____

_____

_____

_____

_____

_____

_____

_____

_____

_____

From *Physical Education Assessment Toolkit* by Liz Giles-Brown, 2006, Champaign, IL: Human Kinetics.

FORM 9.6 **Muscular Strength and Endurance**

Muscular endurance is . . .

Muscular strength is . . .

People with healthy levels of muscular strength and endurance . . .

To improve muscular strength, I can . . .

To improve muscular endurance, I can . . .

Two activities that improve muscular endurance of the abdominal muscles are . . .

Two activities that will improve upper-body strength are . . .

The difference between muscular strength and endurance is . . .

Muscular endurance is the ability to use the muscles many times without getting . . .

People with healthy levels of muscular strength and endurance are more likely to . . .

To produce increases in muscular strength and endurance, the muscles must be . . .

If you want to be able to jump farther, you'll have to overload lower-body muscles by . . .

If you place extra demands on your muscles, those muscles will . . .

If my goal is to increase strength I need to . . .

If my goal is to increase muscular endurance I need to . . .

Two health benefits of maintaining healthful levels of muscular strength and endurance are . . .

Exercise and playing hard help to keep the muscles . . .

Push-ups and curl-ups are examples of exercises that improve . . .

Muscles get stronger when they do more work than they are . . .

When I do muscular strength and endurance exercises I feel . . .

Other open-ended closure statements that can be used to assess students' knowledge and understanding of muscular strength and endurance:

_____

_____

_____

_____

_____

_____

_____

_____

_____

_____

_____

Body Composition

My body is made up of . . .

A healthy amount of fat in my body will . . .

Cardiorespiratory activities help burn fat to use for . . .

People who have a healthful body composition . . .

People who have an unhealthful level of body fat are more likely to . . .

My lean body tissue is made up of . . .

To maintain a healthy body composition, I can choose to . . .

Other open-ended closure statements that can be used to assess students' knowledge and understanding of body composition:

_____

_____

_____

_____

_____

_____

_____

_____

_____

_____

_____

_____

_____

_____

_____

_____

_____

_____

_____

_____

_____

_____

From *Physical Education Assessment Toolkit* by Liz Giles-Brown, 2006, Champaign, IL: Human Kinetics.

FORM 9.8 **Cardiorespiratory Fitness**

Cardiorespiratory fitness is . . .

The inside parts of the body most involved in cardiorespiratory activities are . . .

When I am active, my breathing rate . . .

When I am active, my heart rate . . .

Three changes that take place in my body when I am participating in cardiorespiratory activities are . . .

When I play hard my muscles are working harder and need more . . .

Cardiorespiratory fitness is fitness of the . . .

Three cardiorespiratory activities that I enjoy are . . .

If I make a habit of doing cardiorespiratory activities when I am young, I will . . .

The two body systems that work together during cardiorespiratory activities are . . .

I can tell that I am getting a good cardiorespiratory workout when . . .

To develop healthful levels of cardiorespiratory fitness, I need to participate in them at least . . .

My cardiorespiratory workout should last at least . . .

I should warm up gradually because . . .

I should cool down after exercising hard because . . .

Two other things besides exercising that I can do to keep a strong and healthy heart are . . .

I can tell when a person has healthful levels of cardiorespiratory fitness because he or she . . .

Three reasons why a person would choose to maintain healthful levels of cardiorespiratory fitness are . . .

I can measure the intensity of my cardiorespiratory workout by . . .

Stroke volume is . . .

When I participate in cardiorespiratory endurance activities my stroke volume . . .

When I participate in cardiorespiratory endurance activities the blood flow to my working muscles . . .

When I participate in cardiorespiratory endurance activities the blood flow to my lungs and heart . . .

When I participate in cardiorespiratory endurance activities the blood flow to my digestive organs . . .

When I participate in cardiorespiratory endurance activities my body uses carbohydrates and fats for . . .

Cardiorespiratory activities are those in which people work for longer periods at moderate levels of . . .

When I participate in cardiorespiratory fitness activities my muscles need a continuous supply of . . .

A medium intensity feels like . . .

Two activities that require high levels of cardiorespiratory fitness to be successful are . . .

Two long-term benefits of participating in cardiorespiratory fitness activities are . . .

I can lower my risk factors for heart disease by . . .

Other open-ended closure statements that can be used to assess students' knowledge and understanding of cardiorespiratory endurance:

_____

_____

_____

FORM 9.9 **Health-Related Fitness—Principles of Training**

The components of health-related fitness are . . .

Duration means . . .

Frequency means . . .

Intensity means . . .

To overload means . . .

The progression principle means . . .

If I wanted to improve my flexibility I could apply the overload principle by . . .

If I wanted to improve my flexibility I could apply the progression principle by . . .

If I wanted to improve my muscular endurance I could apply the overload principle by . . .

If I wanted to improve my muscular endurance I could apply the progression principle by . . .

If I wanted to improve my muscular strength I could apply the overload principle by . . .

If I wanted to improve my muscular strength I could apply the progression principle by . . .

If I wanted to improve my cardiorespiratory endurance I could apply the overload principle by . . .

If I wanted to improve my cardiorespiratory endurance I could apply the progression principle by . . .

Other open-ended closure statements that can be used to assess students' knowledge and understanding of health-related fitness principles of training:

_____

_____

_____

_____

_____

_____

_____

_____

_____

_____

_____

_____

_____

_____

_____

From *Physical Education Assessment Toolkit* by Liz Giles-Brown, 2006, Champaign, IL: Human Kinetics.

Skill-Related Fitness

Coordination is . . .

Agility is . . .

Speed is . . .

Power is . . .

Balance is . . .

Reaction time is . . .

If I analyze and understand what components of skill-related fitness are important for activities that I want to participate in, I can . . .

An activity that requires a lot of coordination is . . .

An activity that requires a lot of agility is . . .

An activity that requires a lot of speed is . . .

An activity that requires a lot of power is . . .

An activity that requires a lot of balance is . . .

An activity that requires a quick reaction time is . . .

Three skill-related fitness components are . . .

The skill-related fitness components important for successful participation in (name of activity) are . . .

Other open-ended closure statements that can be used to assess students' knowledge and understanding of skill-related fitness components:

_____

_____

_____

_____

_____

_____

_____

_____

_____

_____

_____

_____

_____

_____

_____

From *Physical Education Assessment Toolkit* by Liz Giles-Brown, 2006, Champaign, IL: Human Kinetics.

Strategy—All Types of Games

For every game or activity there is a . . .

Different types of games have different . . .

Strategy means . . .

I can't really focus on strategy until . . .

Focusing on strategy requires the ability to . . .

One strategy common to all types of games is . . .

Two strategies that I will implement for offensive advantage in (name of activity) games are . . .

Two strategies that I will implement for defensive advantage in (name of activity) games are . . .

Other open-ended closure statements that can be used to assess students' knowledge and understanding of strategies for games:

_____

_____

_____

_____

_____

_____

_____

_____

_____

_____

_____

_____

_____

_____

_____

_____

_____

_____

_____

_____

Strategy—Tag Games

When involved in a tag game I can use my peripheral vision to . . .

Balance and a good ready position are important in tag games because . . .

If I always use the same fake my opponent will . . .

I can use quick changes in speed, direction, and pathway to . . .

To conceal means to . . .

Intent means . . .

In tag games I can conceal my intent by . . .

Other open-ended closure statements that can be used to assess students' knowledge and understanding of strategies for tag games:

_____

_____

_____

_____

_____

_____

_____

_____

_____

_____

_____

_____

_____

_____

_____

_____

_____

_____

_____

_____

_____

_____

From *Physical Education Assessment Toolkit* by Liz Giles-Brown, 2006, Champaign, IL: Human Kinetics.

Strategy—Net Games

Three examples of net games are . . .

Balance and a good ready position are important in net games because . . .

Two offensive strategies that I can use to increase my success in net games are . . .

Two defensive strategies that I can use to increase my success in net games are . . .

Sending the ball or object to the most open area involves . . .

The area that will provide me with the most coverage is . . .

A strategy that I can use in net games that will make it difficult for my opponent to anticipate what I'm going to do is . . .

Communication between teammates in net games is important because . . .

Teammates can help improve each other's performance by . . .

Other open-ended closure statements that can be used to assess students' knowledge and understanding of strategies for net games:

_____

_____

_____

_____

_____

_____

_____

_____

_____

_____

_____

_____

_____

_____

_____

_____

_____

_____

_____

_____

From *Physical Education Assessment Toolkit* by Liz Giles-Brown, 2006, Champaign, IL: Human Kinetics.

Strategy—Target Games

Staying relaxed and confident in target games is important because . . .

Hurrying in target games might . . .

In target games I can get feedback that will help me improve performance from . . .

Mental practice is related to increased performance in target games because . . .

Other open-ended closure statements that can be used to assess students' knowledge and understanding of strategies for target games:

_____

_____

_____

_____

_____

_____

_____

_____

_____

_____

_____

_____

_____

_____

_____

_____

_____

_____

_____

_____

_____

_____

_____

_____

_____

_____

_____

_____

_____

From *Physical Education Assessment Toolkit* by Liz Giles-Brown, 2006, Champaign, IL: Human Kinetics.

Strategy—Invasion Games

Maintaining an athletic ready position in invasion games is important because . . .

I can create open spaces on offense by . . .

I can gain an advantage on offense by . . .

My position on defense should be related to . . .

When I am guarding an opponent I want to . . .

I can increase my chances of intercepting a pass by . . .

In invasion games I can conceal my intent by . . .

When I have control of the ball my priority rules are . . .

Two offensive strategies that I can use in invasion games to increase my success rate are . . .

Two defensive strategies that I can use in invasion games to increase my success rate are . . .

When playing person-to-person defense my primary responsibilities are . . .

When playing a zone defense my primary responsibilities are . . .

When I have the ball on offense I should first look to see if I can . . .

My team can work more efficiently as a unit if . . .

Other open-ended closure statements that can be used to assess students' knowledge and understanding of strategies for invasion games:

_____

_____

_____

_____

_____

_____

_____

_____

_____

_____

_____

_____

_____

_____

_____

_____

Strategy—Fielding Games

Maintaining an athletic ready position in fielding games is important because . . .

When I bat, kick, or throw in fielding games I should try to . . .

Playing a position in fielding games means . . .

Backing up a teammate will . . .

I might be caught unaware in fielding games if . . .

One offensive strategy that I can use in fielding games is . . .

One defensive strategy that I can use in fielding games is . . .

Other open-ended closure statements that can be used to assess students' knowledge and understanding of strategies for fielding games:

_____

_____

_____

_____

_____

_____

_____

_____

_____

_____

_____

_____

_____

_____

_____

_____

_____

_____

_____

_____

_____

_____

From *Physical Education Assessment Toolkit* by Liz Giles-Brown, 2006, Champaign, IL: Human Kinetics.

PART II

Model Units and Ideas on Backward Design

The units presented in chapters 10, 11, and 12 were built using the backward design model of unit development. Planning backward, or beginning with the end, simply means starting at the end. When starting with the end (the assessments in this case), you can develop a clear focus for both yourself and your students. This section provides a brief description of the process. For an in-depth look at this method, I recommend *Understanding by Design*, written by Jay McTighe and Grant Wiggins.

Each of the units in part II follows the same format, providing the following information: unit title, number of lessons, unit summary, unit objectives, unit assessments, and a learning plan with complete descriptive lesson plans. The units serve two purposes. First, they give clear examples of how to develop units using the backward design method of curriculum development. Second, they provide examples of how you can use the assessments provided in this resource within a unit. Each of the three units was developed by identifying answers to the following questions:

I. What should students know, understand, and be able to do by the end of the final lesson? When answering these questions we must focus on what is most important. This is the point at which the results or target of the unit become clear. A common mistake made in physical education is to identify too many objectives for the time available. This practice can cloud the focus for teachers and students and make it difficult to reach any of the objectives. After you narrow the focus to fit the time available, choosing the assessments to use is easier.

2. What methods of assessment can you use to assess the learning? *Physical Education Assessment Toolkit* provides a variety of assessments appropriate to almost any unit in physical education. The assessments chosen to measure learning for the units are examples of some of the templates provided throughout the book and on the accompanying CD-ROM. Unlike traditional ways of planning, backward design requires completion of these two steps before identifying the activities that will help students reach the goals of instruction. Answers to the first two questions lead into the third question.

3. What teaching and learning activities will help students hit the target? When using this method of curriculum development, teachers do not choose activities for their own sake. Activities have a clear connection with the identified targets and assessments chosen. Each lesson plan identifies a concept focus, skill focus, necessary equipment, and a detailed teaching and learning plan.

Something to keep in mind when exploring the process of backward design is that students will benefit from quality instruction and assessment that lead to improved performance. Teaching and assessing for skill development, knowledge, and understanding will help students build a skill and knowledge base that they can apply to an active life. Putting time into careful planning can have positive outcomes in the lives of students and make teaching physical education an extremely rewarding experience.

10 CHAPTER

Force It

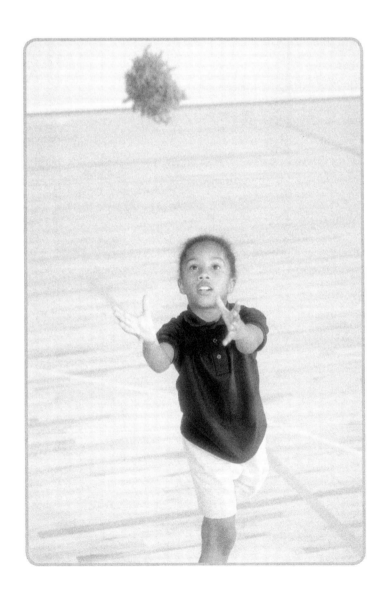

This unit was developed for use with students in grades three through five. During this unit, students will be involved in a variety of tossing, throwing, and catching activities designed to improve mechanics and increase understanding of force production along with basic space concepts for games of invasion. Throughout the unit, you need to offer positive, specific instructional feedback and ask thought-provoking application questions to help all students develop mechanics and understanding. To implement this unit, you will need a variety of balls, beanbags, or other objects safe for tossing, throwing, and catching. Hula hoops, various targets for the walls, pinnies or wristbands, and markers for marking playing areas will also be necessary. You should assign partners for the activity Processing Partners, which is used at various times during the unit.

Unit Objectives

At the end of this unit, students will have had opportunities to develop the following skills:

- Tossing and catching to themselves
- Throwing to a stationary target or partner
- Throwing to a moving target or partner
- Catching a ball thrown to them while stationary
- Catching a ball thrown to them as they move to open spaces
- Using quick changes of speed, direction, and pathway to gain advantage on offense

At the end of this unit, students will have had opportunities to develop and demonstrate knowledge and understanding of the following:

- Mechanics for throwing
- Mechanics for catching

- The amount of force produced can be changed by either changing the movement to include more muscles or increasing the speed of the movement.
- When catching, rebound is reduced by increasing the distance over which the force of the object is absorbed (called absorbing the force).
- In invasion games that include defensive players, moving with quick changes of speed, direction, and pathway when on offense will help gain advantage.

Unit Assessments

The methods of formative knowledge and understanding assessments used during this unit are Force It—Processing Partner Statements (form 10.1) and a peer performance assessment called Force It—Mechanics Check (form 10.2), which gives students individual feedback on throwing mechanics. The summative assessments used to give students opportunities to demonstrate knowledge and understanding of throwing mechanics and force production are Force It—The Alien (form 10.3) and Force It—Pictures (form 10.4). Although students work on other skills and knowledge during the unit, the primary focus for summative assessment purposes is on throwing mechanics and force production concepts. To avoid surprises, give students this information at the beginning of the unit.

Learning Plan

The following lesson progression helps students meet the goals and objectives for this unit, successfully complete the targeted assessments, and have a safe, enjoyable, and educational physical experience.

Lesson #1   Mechanics

CONCEPT FOCUS

Mechanics, force

SKILL FOCUS

Tossing and catching

EQUIPMENT AND MATERIALS

Assorted balls or beanbags that vary in difficulty to toss and catch (ideally, one per student), five or six hoops, CD player and music (optional)

TEACHING AND LEARNING ACTIVITIES

Setup

Place one ball for each student in open spaces around the gym. The balls should be of a type that all students can toss and catch successfully. On the sidelines in hoops or other containers, have a variety of balls in graduated difficulty to toss and catch. As students walk into the gym, instruct them to stand beside the ball of their choice. Having the equipment scattered before students come into the gym will reduce the time needed to distribute equipment.

Warm-Up—You Choose (5 Minutes)

You can use the warm-up activity called You Choose each time you introduce a new skill or piece of equipment. You Choose gives students a chance to be creative and try different tricks and skills that you may not have thought of. When you give students some freedom, they often come up with wonderful new ideas to incorporate in future lessons. This activity also gives you an opportunity to do a quick general skill assessment before getting started.

Rules and Procedures

1. Students must use equipment safely in self-space.

2. If equipment goes out of a student's space, he or she may retrieve it but must return to his or her space before continuing.

3. On the signal to stop, everyone should put his or her ball on the ground and listen for the next set of instructions.

Mechanics and Concept Scramble (5 Minutes)

Use a mechanics review to remind students of the important skill cues that they must use to perform the skill correctly. Students in grades three through five should already be familiar with the mechanics for tossing and catching. Teachers often use various skill cues and key words to help students visualize the correct way of performing the skill. They often have students sit down and listen as they review or go over mechanics. Mechanics and Concept Scramble is a more active way to accomplish this.

Directions

1. On the signal to go (music works well), students move into open spaces, each traveling with a ball with balance and control.

2. When the music stops, students stop and put their balls down.

3. Ask them to complete one of the following sentences: "An important skill cue for catching is . . ." (keep your eyes on the ball, move to get in front of or under the ball, give with the force of the ball, and so on) or "An important skill cue for tossing is . . ." (follow through in the direction you want the ball to go, extend your arm as you toss, use a backswing and follow-through, and so on).

4. Tell students to let you know that they have an answer by tossing and catching their balls in self-space.

5. When most students are tossing and catching, give the signal to stop and ask them to share their answers. You can make a list on chart paper or whiteboard as you receive their answers.

6. Repeat this process as needed to get all the skill cues and force concepts that you are looking for. This procedure prevents students from sitting too long and keeps them engaged in the skill that they should be thinking about. The following list provides examples of open-ended statements that you can use for this activity:

   ▪ If I want to be really good at catching I should . . .
   ▪ If I want the ball to go where I want it to go, I need to . . .
   ▪ Two important things to remember about tossing are . . .
   ▪ Two important things to remember about catching are . . .

Graduating Difficulty (10 to 15 Minutes)

Organize the balls on the sideline so that from left to right they increase in difficulty for tossing and catching. In this individual activity, students work at their own pace.

Directions

1. Tell students that they will be working on their tossing and catching skills to graduate to balls that are more difficult to toss and catch. While working in self-space, they need to think about the important skill cues for tossing and catching.

2. Each student must start with the balls that you have designated for easiest catching. To graduate from one ball to the next, a student must be able to toss to a high level 10 times in a row without missing.

3. When a student completes 10 consecutive tosses and catches with a ball from the first hoop, he or she returns it to its hoop and gets one from the next hoop. Note: Do a quick demonstration to let students know what height you expect them to toss to while performing this task. The height will vary depending on grade level.

4. At the end of this activity, instruct students to choose a ball that they believe they can catch most consistently and place it on the ground in their self-space to get ready for a fun tossing and catching game. Talk about what *consistent* means in this situation.

Note: This is an excellent place to remind students of the virtues they can practice during this activity. Honesty would be a key virtue to reinforce.

Power-Up Tag (10 to 15 Minutes)

Power-Up Tag combines a tag activity with tossing and catching practice and is a fun way for students to continue working on consistency.

Directions

1. When all students are ready and have chosen a ball, tell them that they will have a chance to practice before the game starts.

2. Place five or six hoops in open spaces within the playing area before beginning. When the music starts, students practice their best tossing and catching while moving through general space. They should travel at a speed that will allow them to toss and catch successfully. If students discover that they have chosen a ball that will not allow them to be consistently successful, they should choose a different ball. After the game starts they must stick with their chosen ball.

3. After everyone is set, stop the music and give the instructions. In this game all students are taggers. When the music starts again, students move into open spaces, tossing and catching. At the same time, they try to get close enough to other players so that they can tag them gently. If a player is tagged or drops his or her ball, he or she must repower before reentering the game. To repower, the player must move to an open hoop and toss and catch to a high level 10 times in a row. The hoops are used so that students can work on their follow-through and gain consistency in tossing straight up. The hoops also let other players know that a person has been tagged and is temporarily out of the tag game. Set out as many hoops as needed. After tossing and catching 10 times in a row, the student may reenter the game.

Variations

■ Have the tagged players or players who have dropped a ball stand in a high-five position and become free if another person gives them a high five.

■ A tagged person or player who has dropped the ball must come to you and answer a question about tossing and catching mechanics.

■ A tagged player or player who drops the ball sits where he or she is tagged. The player tosses and catches until the next round. In this variation a round should last for only about a minute so that players do not sit too long.

Closure (1 to 2 Minutes)

Revisit the questions asked during Mechanics and Concept Scramble. You can use some of the posters mentioned in chapter 8 as visual points of reference. Homework for the week is to toss and catch at least 50 times each day while focusing on the important skill cues.

Lesson #2 Challenge Me

CONCEPT FOCUS

Level, applying nonlocomotor movements

SKILL FOCUS

Tossing and catching

EQUIPMENT AND MATERIALS

Assorted balls or beanbags or tossing objects (one per student is ideal), five or six hoops, CD player and music (optional)

TEACHING AND LEARNING ACTIVITIES

Setup

Have a variety of balls from the previous lesson available on the sideline of the activity area. Scatter five or six hoops in the activity area. As students walk into the gym instruct them to choose a ball that they can be successful with, find a self-space while avoiding the hoops, and practice tossing and catching.

Warm-Up (3 to 5 Minutes)

When all students are situated tell them that they will warm up with a variation of the Power-Up Tag game that they played during the last class. Give quick instructions for the variation you choose and then play for two to three minutes.

One on One (8 to 10 Minutes)

After you teach it, you can use One on One, a skill practice activity, at any time and with any skill. As with many other activities, students can be doing a targeted fitness activity and listening to directions at the same time. If you have established fitness routines as described in chapter 1 (flexibility or muscular endurance), students could be performing one as you give directions for this activity.

Directions

1. On the signal to go, students face another person, each with his or her own ball. Together they say, "One, two, ready, go . . ." On "Go," both students begin performing the individual skill (in this case, tossing and catching).

2. They continue until one student drops his or her ball. When that happens they shake hands and say, "Good game."

3. The student able to perform the skill longer wins the round. Both students move to a designated area (possibly the center circle) and find new partners to challenge.

4. Students may not turn down a challenge. As with other activities in which students will be working with many partners, remind them of the effect of body language when working with others.

Challenging Catches (8 to 10 Minutes)

Challenging Catches is an activity that gives students opportunities to practice catching in different places around the body.

Directions

1. Tell students that during the next activity they will practice catching in different ways. They will begin with a ball in an open space.

2. Tell them that when someone tosses or throws them a ball, it doesn't always go directly to their hands so they will need some practice catching at different levels and places around the body. Tell them to listen to the questions and answer with their movement.

3. While moving throughout the room ask the following questions to give feedback as you observe students' movement answers.

   - Can you toss to a high level and catch in a medium level?
   - Can you toss to a high level and catch at a low level?
   - Can you toss to a high level and time a jump to catch in a high level?
   - Can you toss the ball so that you have to twist to catch?
   - Can you toss the ball so that you have to reach to the side to catch?
   - As you catch are you remembering to absorb force so that no rebound occurs?

Sequence the Skills (8 to 10 Minutes)

During this activity, students will develop a catching sequence that combines different levels and body actions.

Directions

1. Instruct students to design a tossing and catching sequence that incorporates four different catches. As a group, brainstorm the possibilities. Possible answers are low level, medium level, stretching out, jumping to catch, reaching to catch, and twisting to catch.

2. Write the responses on a whiteboard or flip chart so that all can refer to the list.

3. Tell students that they have about 10 minutes to complete a sequence. When they finish, they are to practice the sequence and memorize it so that they can perform it consistently.

4. As students work, travel around observing and giving appropriate feedback. When students have completed a sequence and are in the process of practicing, have them stop to listen for the next set of instructions.

   Note: Skill sequences are a great way for students to practice skills and use some creativity. If students learn a process for sequence or routine development on an individual basis, they can later apply that process when working in groups. One successful way of doing that is to teach students to organize and practice their moves one at a time. They choose the first skill and practice it. After mastering the first skill, they add the second skill and practice the skills together, using a smooth transition. They follow this process until they can perform all their moves, never adding a new move until they have refined the previous moves. An analogy that often works well to get students to think about smooth transitions is the image of butter melting into warm bread or chocolate chips melting into a cookie as it bakes. This visual image gets them to think about melting one movement into another, therefore making the transition from one movement to another very smooth. Having them visualize gymnastics, dance, or ice-skating routines also helps them see the difference between smooth and choppy transitions.

Performance (5 to 10 Minutes)

During these one-on-one performances, students get a chance to perform their sequences for their classmates.

Directions

1. Assign partners to begin the activity. One student performs, and one is the audience. Here, students have an opportunity to focus on the skills of being good audience members and good performers.

2. Each student should perform his or her sequence three times in a row and then bow to let his or her audience know that he or she is finished. The observer then applauds and offers one piece of positive specific feedback. Partners then switch roles.

3. After both partners have performed and received feedback, they move to a designated area and find a new partner to repeat the process. If students aren't accustomed to giving and receiving feedback and are unsure about what it means to be objective, they will need some instruction here.

Closure (2 Minutes)

Have students stand facing their processing partners. Ask them to come to consensus on how to complete the following statement and to sit down to signal that they are finished: "Two activities in which I have seen the participants catch by twisting, reaching, or jumping are . . ." (basketball, football, Frisbee, softball, baseball, lacrosse, and so on). Ideally, all partnerships will be able share their answers, but sometimes you just won't have enough time. After someone shares an answer, ask others to raise their hands if they came up with the same answer. That way everyone contributes in some way. As students leave the gym tell them that their homework is to practice their sequence for a game of One on One, with sequences at the beginning of the next class.

Lesson #3   Finding Force

CONCEPT FOCUS

Force concepts

SKILL FOCUS

Tossing, catching, throwing

EQUIPMENT AND MATERIALS

A variety of balls or objects safe for tossing and catching (one of each kind per student), one polyspot per student, CD player and music (optional)

TEACHING AND LEARNING ACTIVITIES

Setup

Have a variety of balls, beanbags, or objects for tossing and catching set out on the side of the activity area.

Warm-Up (2 to 3 Minutes)

As students walk into the gym instruct them to pick up the ball that they used for their sequences during the last class, find an open space, and practice their sequences to get ready for One on One.

One on One (5 Minutes)

Students play One on One (instructions in lesson #2), but this time they must use their individual catching sequences.

Skill Quota (10 Minutes)

This is another skill activity that you can teach once and then use for a variety of skills. Balls for this activity should be those that everyone in the class can be successful with. Students will have a range of partners, and your choice of balls will have an effect on their success.

Note: Remind students of the virtues that they need to practice when working with others and the roles that they might play when working with classmates who are less skilled, of equal ability, or more skilled.

Directions

1. During Skill Quota, students begin with a partner and must cooperate to meet a quota (number of catches) that you set to score points.

2. Each time a partnership meets a quota each person gets 10 points, moves to a designated area to get a new partner, and attempts to meet the quota again with a new partner.

3. You can change the quota or skill any time during the activity. During this game the skill is partner tossing and catching, and the quota starts at six catches in a row. You can challenge students to reach a certain number of points within a designated period.

4. As students participate in this activity, move around the gym and give feedback according to the skill cues for tossing underhand. Focus on the arm swing, the step forward, and the follow-through.

5. While students work, place spots in the area as described in the next activity to shorten transition time from this activity to the next.

6. After about 10 minutes of play have students sit down with the partners whom they are working with and listen to the next set of directions. If you wish, at this time you can have students share high scores and what they did to ensure success.

7. Play another round, having students use the overhead throw instead of the underhand toss. During this round, watch for common mistakes such as stepping forward with the same side of the body as the throwing hand. Offer students feedback that will improve performance.

Finding the Force (10 to 15 Minutes)

The purpose of this activity is for students to discover how they can change their movement when the amount of force necessary changes. Ultimately, they need to know that several things influence how much or how little force the body can produce. They need to know how preparatory movements (backswing when tossing), speed of movement, and the number of muscles used (twisting and stepping forward in opposition with an overhand throw) affect the amount of force that they can produce. Understanding these concepts will help students to improve control in the performance of many skills.

Students will be working with partners to think about force production as they work on tossing, throwing, and catching skills.

Directions

1. Arrange the students so that partners are facing each other, standing on spots or markers that are located at gradually increasing distances from one another as the line extends from one pair of partners to the next. The first partnership stands on spots that are fairly close together,

and the last partnership stands on spots that are the farthest apart. When set up and ready to go, students resemble a giant V.

2. Tell students that they are going to work together to move the ball back and forth without letting it hit the ground. They will need to choose the skill that creates just the right amount of force and allows the partners to catch the ball successfully at each distance.

3. Question students about mechanics for catching and the concept of force absorption. After a minute or so, stop the action and have students rotate to the next set of spots. The students who began standing at the farthest distance apart run to the beginning, where the spots are the shortest distance apart. Tell them as they work that they need to be thinking about how their movement changes so that they can get the ball to their partners each time they move to a new set of spots.

4. Interject questions directed toward those changes after each round.

5. Stop the action at various intervals and ask partners to raise their hands if they beat their previous score.

6. Follow the same procedure until all partnerships have had a chance to try all distances. Then have students identify the change in body action that occurs when the distance increases from short to long.

Closure (2 Minutes)

Have students stand facing their processing partners. Ask them to come to consensus on how to complete the following statement and to sit down to signal that they are finished: "Two things I can do to change the amount of force that I produce when throwing or tossing are . . ." (increase or decrease the speed of the movement, use more muscles, larger backswing, bigger step, more twist with the throw, and so on). Ideally, all groups will be able to share their answers, but sometimes you just won't have enough time. Ask other groups to raise their hands if they came up with the same answers as those who do share. That way everyone gets to contribute in some way.

Lesson #4   Force and Accuracy

CONCEPT FOCUS

Accuracy, follow-through

SKILL FOCUS

Tossing, throwing, and catching

EQUIPMENT AND MATERIALS

One soft, no-bounce ball per student, 10 to 12 targets for the walls, polyspots, one peer overhand throw assessment Force It—Mechanics Check (form 10.2) per student, one pencil per student, CD player and music (optional)

TEACHING AND LEARNING ACTIVITIES

Setup

In open spaces around the room, place soft, easy-to-catch balls that are heavy enough to throw from a distance and that are OK to throw against the walls. Place the balls so that students can walk to a ball as they enter class. Yarn balls or knit balls work well. Tape to or hang on the wall 10 to 12 targets (half as many targets as the number of students in your largest class), evenly distributed around the room. Have pencils and peer assessment sheets for the overhand throw ready for student use.

Warm-Up (2 to 3 Minutes)

As music plays, students use a ball in self-space with control and balance until everyone is ready. Ask them if they can come up with tossing and catching tricks that they can practice. Move and say things like, "I see someone tossing under her leg and catching . . . I see someone tossing, clapping, and catching . . . I see someone tossing, touching the ground, and catching . . . I see someone tossing, turning 360 degrees, and catching . . . I see (fill in anything interesting that you're seeing)." This method will give students ideas about what they might try.

Step-Back Throwing Assessment (8 to 10 Minutes)

This assessment activity involves students in peer assessment on throwing mechanics.

Directions

1. Set up students in partnerships and instruct them to find a space in which they face a section of the wall. They need one pencil and two peer assessment sheets (Force It—Mechanics Check, form 10.2) for the overhand throw. Ask them to recall the correct mechanics for throwing. They begin by standing five steps from the wall that they are facing.

2. On the signal to start, students throw toward the wall, attempting to use the right amount of force to hit it. If they hit the wall they get to step back. Be sure they know that they don't have to concentrate on hitting anything on the wall; they just need to hit it. If they reach a point where the thrown ball does not reach the wall, they need to work from that distance until they can find the force that will allow them to be successful. When they are able to hit the wall, they may move back.

3. As one partner works and steps back, the other partner watches the movement and checks the appropriate items on the peer assessment sheet. On your signal, students sit down and the assessor shares what he or she observed by going over the checklist. Partners then switch roles.

   Thread—personal and social interactions: When students do peer assessments you need to remind them about what being objective means. They must learn to look at the movement itself and detach it from the person. Someone who is objective will perform a fair assessment of both a best friend and someone whom he or she might not know well.

Processing Partners (1 to 2 Minutes)

Have students stand facing their processing partners. Ask them to come to consensus on how to complete the following statement and to sit down to signal that they are finished: "In many throwing and catching activities using the correct amount of force is important. Something else that is sometimes equally as important is . . ." (accuracy). If only a few groups are sitting to signal that they have an answer, give the class this clue: "It begins with the letter A." As students talk with each other, move around the room and place polyspots at different distances from each target. Each polyspot should have one ball on top of it. Call on groups for answers. If you call on one group and they have the correct answer, ask others to raise their hands if they came up with the same answer.

Thread—consensus decision making: Whenever you have time to help students improve their ability to make decisions with another person, briefly review the class procedure for consensus decision making. This skill does not come naturally for all people. The more guidance students receive and the more practice they get, the more they will improve and the more smoothly your classes will run. Everybody wins! Remember to use the vocabulary so that using the correct terms becomes second nature.

Target Practice (15 to 18 Minutes)

Target Practice gives students a chance to work on both accuracy and force. Students will need new partners before you begin.

Directions

1. Tell the class that they will be combining what they know about force production with the need for accuracy as they practice hitting targets from different distances. Have them remind you of the correct mechanics for tossing and throwing. Ask them how the follow-through will help them be more accurate.

2. On the signal to go they move with their partners to a target, where they will find one ball and one polyspot. The goal is to hit the target, using correct mechanics without stepping over the polyspot. In turn, each partner gets two attempts. For every hit, the partnership earns 100 points.

3. When the music stops or on a signal, students place the ball on the spot and move to the next target. This station activity will allow you to talk with all students and offer positive, specific instructional feedback on their throwing and tossing skills.

Note: Teachers often pay little attention to how students form partnerships. When students choose partners on a regular basis, one or two students whom nobody wants to be with are guaranteed to be left standing, often the same one or two students each time. What must that do to their self-esteem? This experience can be awful, and it sends a definite message: "Nobody wants to be with me. I'm not good at this." We do not want students to feel that way about themselves in physical activity settings. They will forever attach those negative feelings to physical education class and may transfer them to other physical activity settings. Students need to experience positive emotions in physical education. Therefore, you should probably assign partners when starting a new activity. With some fast-action activities that include a lot of partner scrambles, it's part of the activity to have students choose partners, but when you're starting a new activity and the attention is on getting a partner, the safest idea is to assign partners yourself.

Closure (1 to 2 Minutes)

Have students stand facing their processing partners. Ask them to come to consensus on how to complete the following statement and to sit down to signal that they are finished: "One activity in which participants need to be able to throw using force and accuracy is . . ." Ideally, all groups will be able to share their answers, but sometimes you just won't have enough time. Ask other groups to raise their hands if they came up with the same answers as those who do share. That way everyone gets to contribute in some way. Tell students that their homework is to practice throwing for accuracy at least three times before their next physical education class.

Lesson #5 Putting It Together

CONCEPT FOCUS

Using quick changes of speed, direction, and pathway

SKILL FOCUS

Tossing or throwing to a moving target

EQUIPMENT AND MATERIALS

One soft ball appropriate for successful tossing and catching for each student, markers for creating grids (square spaces in which separate games will take place)

TEACHING AND LEARNING ACTIVITIES

Warm-Up (5 Minutes)

During some of the activities that follow, students will need to move at different speeds and in different pathways. This activity will get them thinking about these space concepts. As students enter the gym ask them to find an open space. When all students are in open spaces tell them that you are going to play some music and that they should move into open spaces. On your signal they must stop with good balance. On each signal ask them to respond to one of the following statements:

- Move into open spaces using straight pathways.
- Move into open spaces using curved pathways.
- Move into open spaces using zigzag pathways.
- Move into open spaces using change of speed.
- Move into open spaces using change of speed and change of pathway.
- Imagine that someone is playing defense against you and doesn't want you to get the ball. Use change of speed, direction, and pathway along with some fakes to get to the open spaces.

Processing Partners (1 to 2 Minutes)

Have students stand facing their processing partners. Ask them to come to consensus on how to complete the following statement and to sit down to signal that they are finished: "Three activities in which the players must use quick changes of speed, direction, and pathway in order to move into open spaces are . . ." Ideally, all groups will be able to share their answers, but sometimes you just won't have enough time. Ask other groups to raise their hands if they came up with the same answers as those who do share. That way everyone gets to contribute in some way.

Musical Toss Tag (5 Minutes)

Musical Toss Tag is a high-energy skill practice activity. Students start with their processing partners from the last activity.

Directions

1. When the music starts, partners begin tossing and catching from locations a short distance apart. When the music stops, whoever is holding the ball or about to catch the ball is a tagger. The person without the ball is a runner. All taggers run and try to tag anyone without a

ball except their own partners. As the game continues the number of people a person can tag decreases because he or she cannot ever tag anyone who has been his or her partner at any point during the game.

2. When a person with a ball tags a runner, the tagger and runner begin tossing and catching with each other. When the music starts again, anyone who does not have a new partner must team up and begin tossing and catching. They listen for the next round to begin while they continue to toss and catch.

3. Instruct students to use quick changes of speed, direction, and pathway to avoid being tagged.

Partner Pass Practice (15 to 20 Minutes)

During Partner Pass Practice, students will have opportunities to practice different ways to move into open spaces to catch a ball. Using polyspots or cones, section off the gym into squares or rectangles of space in which you will assign students to work.

Directions

1. Assign partners and then distribute them among the designated spaces. Avoid placing more than three partnerships in any one space.

2. Have partners begin by throwing and tossing to each other while they are stationary. Remind them to focus on using correct mechanics. Use this time to check mechanics and offer feedback.

3. After a few minutes, change the task. Tell students that in most activities involving throwing and catching, the person receiving the ball is not standing still. He or she is moving to get away from defenders by using quick changes of speed, direction, and pathway. In this phase of the activity, the person with the ball remains stationary while the receiver cuts to open spaces to receive the pass on the go. Ask this question: "What has to change about the throw or toss to make a complete pass?" (The throw has to lead or be out in front of the runner so that he or she does not have to stop to catch.) Continue with the activity, stopping and giving positive, specific instructional feedback as needed.

Complete Passes—No Defense (6 to 10 Minutes)

In Complete Passes—No Defense, students stay in the same space. This is a lead-up for another activity that students will participate in during the next class period.

Directions

1. Tell students that they will be practicing the same skills they did before except that now they must complete three passes in a row to score.

2. For every three passes completed they receive 10 points. Groups try to beat their highest score during each round of play. For a pass to count as a completed pass, the passer must remain stationary while the receiver uses quick changes of speed, direction, and pathway to move to the open spaces.

3. If a receiver drops the ball, partners must begin counting again from one. This activity works well with music. Put the music on for one minute of play and then stop it. As students play, watch for those who slip back into standing and catching instead of moving to the open spaces.

4. After each minute of play, tell students that they have 30 seconds to confer with their partners and come up with a strategy to beat their previous score.

Variations

■ Have students change partners within their space after each round of play.

■ Change the number of passes that partnerships must complete to earn a score.

■ Have students work in groups of three instead of two.

Closure

Have students stand facing their processing partners. Ask them to come to consensus on how to complete the following statement and to sit down to signal that they are finished: "One important thing to remember when throwing to moving partners is to . . . " (throw the ball ahead of them so that they don't have to stop and catch, lead them with the pass, throw the ball to where they are going instead of where they are). Ideally, all groups will be able to share their answers, but sometimes you just won't have enough time. Ask other groups to raise their hands if they came up with the same answers as those who do share. That way everyone gets to contribute in some way. Tell students that their homework is to play catch with somebody each day for five minutes.

Lesson #6   A Little Competition

CONCEPT FOCUS

Accuracy

SKILL FOCUS

Throwing, tossing, catching

EQUIPMENT AND MATERIALS

One soft ball appropriate for successful tossing and catching for each student, markers for creating grids (square spaces in which separate games will take place)

TEACHING AND LEARNING ACTIVITIES

Setup

Place balls on the sideline. Choose balls that all students can be successful with.

Warm-Up

Assign students to partnerships or groups of three and have them set up in their spaces. Two groups should occupy each space. Tell them to warm up their muscles by practicing throwing and catching with the thrower standing still and the catcher moving to the open spaces. To use time efficiently, after a few minutes instruct students to perform one of their individual fitness routines (see chapter 2 for more information) while listening to the next set of directions.

Complete Passes With Defense

This activity is a continuation of Complete Passes—No Defense from the last lesson. Students will again try to complete three passes, but this time the other group in their space will attempt to intercept passes by playing person-to-person defense. The amount of instruction required for the defensive portion of this activity will depend on students' experience.

Directions

1. One team in each playing area begins on offense. Each time the offensive team completes three passes they score 10 points. That team remains on offense until you give the signal to switch.

2. If a defensive player intercepts the ball, he or she places it on the ground and gets into position for play to resume. One of the offensive players picks up the ball and starts play again.

3. After two or three minutes of play, signal students to switch offensive and defensive roles.

4. Each time a group is on offense, they try to beat their previous score. Stress that when players are on defense, they must play person to person and cannot double-team.

5. After a while, have the teams rotate to another space so that they play against another team.

Note: While giving instructions be sure to remind students of the skills and concepts that they will need to apply to be successful. A good way to do this is to ask leading questions while giving instructions. Another good time to use this technique and offer feedback would be when you stop play to have students switch from offense to defense and vice versa.

Closure (1 to 2 Minutes)

Partners from the last activity stand facing each other. Ask them to share two things that they did well while working together and one thing that they need to improve.

Lesson #7   Skill Applications

CONCEPT FOCUS

Force, accuracy

SKILL FOCUS

Tossing, throwing, catching

EQUIPMENT AND MATERIALS

Many soft knit, foam, or yarn balls (the more the better); scrimmage vests, wristbands, or some other method of identifying teams for half the class; markers to designate a centerline; four hoops (two of one color and two of another); CD player and music (optional)

TEACHING AND LEARNING ACTIVITIES

Setup

Have balls available on the sidelines as students enter the room.

Warm-Up (5 to 6 Minutes)

As students enter the gym, assign partners and ask them to find a space where they can throw and catch while focusing on correct mechanics. Organize the class so that each person is facing his or her partner with the centerline between them. In the absence of a centerline, use markers to establish one. The objective of this warm-up game is to see how far apart partners can move without dropping the ball. They begin close together and toss the ball back and forth. After each partner catches one toss from the other, they each take one step backward and try again. As they move farther apart they must change the movement to produce enough force to get the ball to each other. If the ball touches the ground they must start back at the centerline.

Catch It—Keep It (20 to 25 Minutes)

This game works in a progressive manner with a series of steps. As you teach it, you add different rules. Divide the class in half. Have each group sit in a line in one half of the gym.

Directions

1. Divide the playing space with a line in the center. Cones or polyspots will work if there is no center dividing line.

2. Give one team vests or wristbands so that they can be easily identified. Ask both teams to sit in a circle. Their task is to divide themselves into two equal groups by using the consensus decision-making process.

3. After they have done that, instruct half of each team to cross the centerline and sit down. Half of each team will then be on each side of the line. Each team has divided itself into two groups that will work together as a team.

4. Place a hoop for each team at the back of each playing side of the playing area (four hoops total) and scatter the balls throughout the gym. Each team must know the color of the hoop that they will be using. Ideally, the color of the hoops will correspond with the color of the scrimmage vests or wristbands.

5. Tell students that they will be playing a game that has a series of steps that make it more challenging as they progress. Then give the instructions for step 1.

Step 1

Introduce this activity to students as one in which they will be applying all the skills and concepts that they have worked on during this unit.

Directions

1. Groups see how many balls they can catch and keep.

2. The opposing team may not interfere with a team's efforts at this point.

3. If a player throws or tosses a ball across the line and a teammate catches it, that person takes the ball and places it in his or her team's hoop on that side of the room. The only major rule in this first simple step of the activity is that a ball on the ground cannot be kept (or placed in a hoop).

4. Players must catch the ball in the air. Players on the opposing team may not interfere at this stage of the game.

5. A player holding a ball can only pivot. He or she may not move into general space.

6. Receivers can move into the open spaces.

7. Once a ball is placed in a hoop located in the back of the playing area, it may not be taken out.

8. Have students play for about two minutes. Then stop the action and clear up any confusion or answer any questions that students may have.

9. Have the two halves of each team count the balls, meet in the middle, and add up their total score. Their objective in the next round is to beat their previous score. Play a couple rounds, stop the action, and move to step 2.

Step 2

During this phase, students play defense as well as offense. Students remain on the same side of the playing area. Scatter the balls around again. Game play continues as before, but now players on the opposing team can intercept passes. Stress that no body contact is permitted. At this point, ask students what they can do to get to open spaces (move using quick changes of speed, direction, and pathway to get into the open spaces). Play a few rounds, with teams attempting to beat their previous scores. As students play this game, watch for correct mechanics and how students are using their bodies to produce and absorb force. Give appropriate positive, specific instructional feedback. Jot down the composition of the teams so that you have a list for the next class period in case students forget.

Closure

Have students stand facing their processing partners. Ask them to come to consensus on how to complete the following statement and to sit down to signal that they are finished: "Three skills that helped me be successful during the game today are . . ." (changing speed and direction quickly, catching, throwing, moving into open spaces, throwing to a moving partner, and so on). Ideally, all groups will be able to share their answers, but sometimes you just won't have enough time. Ask other groups to raise their hands if they came up with the same answers as those who do share. That way everyone gets to contribute in some way. Tell students just before they leave class that the game they started playing today has several more steps and to be ready for more action during the next class. Their homework is to remember who is on their team.

Lesson #8 Step It Up!

CONCEPT FOCUS

Defense, offense, force production, accuracy, creating space

SKILL FOCUS

Throwing; catching; using change of speed, direction, and pathway

EQUIPMENT AND MATERIALS

Many soft knit, foam, or yarn balls (the more balls the better); scrimmage vests, wristbands, or some other method of identifying teams for half the class; markers to designate a centerline; four hoops (two of one color and two of another); CD player and music (optional)

TEACHING AND LEARNING ACTIVITIES

Setup

Set up the gym the way it was for the last round of Catch It—Keep It. Scatter the balls and place two hoops at the back of each playing space.

Warm-Up (3 to 5 Minutes)

As students come into the gym have them each get two balls from the floor. As the music plays, students should experiment with different ways to toss and catch two balls at the same time.

Catch It–Keep It (25 to 30 Minutes)

Organize students into their teams from the last class. Have one team wear the pinnies, scrimmage vests, or wristbands. Give them one minute to use consensus decision making to divide their team into two groups. Review the rules for step 2 from the previous lesson and play one round.

Step 3

During step 3, one team is on offense and the other team plays defense. The teams change roles after a designated period. Make sure that all students understand this major change in the structure of the activity.

Directions

1. The job of the offensive team is to catch as many balls as they can and place them in their hoops. They are playing offense only and don't have to worry about trying to intercept balls thrown by the other team because the job of the other team is to play defense only. In step 2, teams were playing both offense and defense at the same time.

2. The defensive team plays person-to-person defense to intercept or block passes. If a defensive player intercepts a ball during this step, he or she places it on the ground and continues to play defense.

3. Another notable change is that while on offense both the thrower and the catcher may use quick changes of speed, direction, and pathway to move to get open. Before, only the catcher could move, and the thrower could only pivot from where he or she picked up the ball. You may need to demonstrate how these changes will affect the action.

4. After the first round of step 3 have the offensive team count the number of balls that they were able to keep. Then have the offensive team switch to defense and the defensive team play offense. Each team should play offense and defense an equal number of times.

5. After every two rounds briefly question students about mechanics, choice of skill, force production, and use of space.

Step 4

During this step the game itself stays the same, but you introduce the team plan.

Directions

1. Instruct students to sit with their teams in a circle formation for consensus decision making. Tell them that they have two to three minutes to come up with a plan. Observe how the groups work and offer feedback targeted toward the consensus decision-making process.

2. After they have had a chance to come up with a plan, have them split up and play more rounds.

Closure (1 to 2 Minutes)

Give the students feedback on the strategy plans and tell them that during the next class period they will participate in some assessments and skill centers. For homework, students should review all the skill cues for throwing and what they can do to change the amount of force that they produce.

Lesson #9   Assessment Time

CONCEPT FOCUS

Force production, mechanics

SKILL FOCUS

Throwing, catching, tossing

EQUIPMENT AND MATERIALS

Force It—The Alien (form 10.3) and Force It—Pictures (form 10.4) assessment sheets for each student, one pencil per student, one clipboard per student, one jump rope per student, a variety of balls for experimenting, equipment that will be used during the next unit

TEACHING AND LEARNING ACTIVITIES

Setup

Set up the following list of centers before students enter the gym. A brief list of ideas follows. You can use other centers as well.

1. Force It—The Alien (form 10.3)—assessment sheets, pencils, and clipboards

2. Force It—Pictures (form 10.4)—assessment sheets, pencils, and clipboards

3. Trick center—a variety of balls for students to experiment with

4. Partner center—a variety of balls for work with partners

5. Cardio center—jump ropes for students to work on cardiorespiratory fitness

6. Primer—equipment that will be used during the next unit to prime students and get them interested

Directions

1. As students enter the gym tell them that today they will have an assessment center class and that they need to sit on the sideline and listen carefully to instructions.

2. Go over the instructions for each assessment sheet and answer any questions that students may have. Tell students that they may choose which assessment they want to do first.

3. Before they begin working on their assessment sheets, give directions for each center. Tell them that when they finish both assessment sheets, they should hand them to you. They may then visit any of the centers. They decide how to spend the remainder of their time. This is a great example of the power of choice.

4. Students who don't finish their assessment sheets can finish them for homework or you can give them a few minutes at the beginning of the following class period.

5. After you correct the assessments, return them, go over possible correct answers, and tell any student who has a question about how you scored his or her paper to see you directly after class.

Force It—Processing Partner Statements

An important skill cue for catching is . . .

An important skill cue for tossing is . . .

Important things that I need to remember if I want to be good at catching are . . .

When I'm getting ready to throw I should . . .

After I release the ball I should . . .

I can absorb the force of the object that I'm trying to catch by . . .

Two activities in which I have seen participants catch by twisting, reaching, or jumping are . . .

Two things that I can do to change the amount of force I produce when throwing or tossing are . . .

One activity in which participants need to be able to throw using force and accuracy is . . .

Two important things to remember when throwing to a moving partner are . . .

Three skill cues that helped me be successful during the game today are . . .

FORM 10.2 **Force It—Mechanics Check**

Performer's Name _____ **Assessor's Name** _____

SKILL—THROWING

Directions: Watch your classmate perform the skill and check the skill cues that you see him or her performing consistently.

_____ **1.** Always begins by standing side to the target

_____ **2.** Gets ready to throw by bringing the ball down and back in a curved pathway

_____ **3.** Steps forward with a twisting motion on the opposite foot

_____ **4.** Follows through to complete the motion

Force It—The Alien

Name _____ **Date** _____

Directions: An alien landed in our gym and watched as we practiced <u>throwing</u>. The alien had never seen this skill performed before but noticed that some students were successful and some were having difficulty. What are three things that the alien might have seen the successful students doing that the others were not?

1. _____

_____

_____

_____

2. _____

_____

_____

_____

3. _____

_____

_____

_____

Assessment: Your work will be scored according to the criteria in the following rubric. Use this information to self-assess your work before you hand it in.

4	Excellent work! You went above and beyond!	Three correct, complete, specific skill cues are provided. Artwork, specific examples, or details that support answers are included.
3	Good work. Everything is here!	Three correct, complete, specific skill cues are provided.
2	Good attempt. Just a few things are missing. Would you like to give it another try?	At least two correct, complete, specific skill cues are provided.
1	Let's be sure that you understand. I recommend that you try this one again. See me for more explanation.	Fewer than two complete, correct, specific skill cues are provided.

FORM 10.4 **Force It—Pictures**

Name _____ **Date** _____

Use drawings (diagrams) and labels to illustrate <u>how you can use the body to produce force when throwing a ball for distance</u>.

Assessment: Your work will be scored according to the criteria in the following rubric. Use this information to self-assess your work before you hand it in.

4	Excellent work! You went above and beyond!	The response illustrates the concepts specified in the directions. Labels support the illustrations.
3	Good work. Everything is here!	The response illustrates the concepts specified in the directions. Most labels support the illustrations.
2	Good attempt. Just a few things are missing. Would you like to give it another try?	Part of the response illustrates the concepts specified in the directions. Some labels support the illustrations.
1	Let's be sure that you understand. I recommend that you try this one again. See me for more explanation.	Little of the response illustrates the concepts specified in the directions. Labels are inaccurate or missing.

11

CHAPTER

Fly, Birdie, Fly

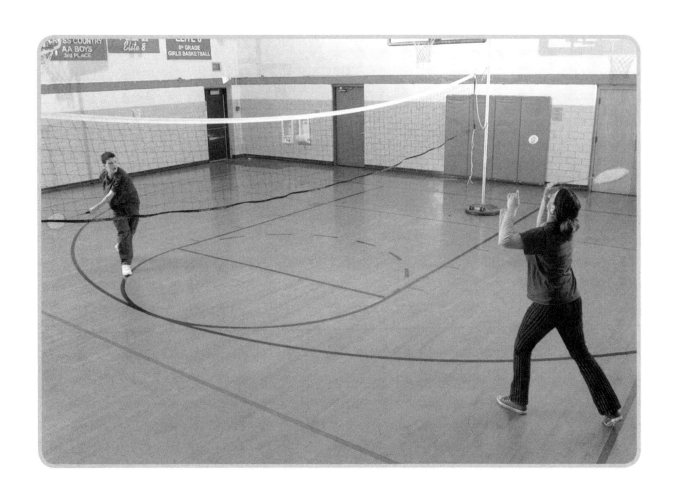

This unit was designed for use with students in grades six through eight but could certainly be used with higher levels. During this unit, students will be involved in a variety of lessons designed to teach the basics of badminton. The badminton serve, clears, smash, drive, and block will be the skill focus. The concept focus is trajectory, angle of impact, and strategies used in net games. The unit begins with students involved in cooperative and competitive skill activities and progresses with a modified ladder tournament with teams using their skills to compete for the top rung of the ladder. This unit offers an excellent opportunity to focus on the value of quality competition and practicing virtues during physical activity. The equipment necessary to implement the unit is one badminton racket per student, three to four birdies per student, one playing court with net and net standards for every four students (you can use volleyball standards to support badminton nets), CD player and music, and one pencil per student.

A unique teaching strategy that you can experiment with during this unit is the purposeful use of a specific type of music to bring about a desired result. Music creates a clear signal for beginning and ending activity, and it can serve as a motivator in many situations. During the course of the unit, Caribbean or steel band music is used to help foster a smoother swing.

Unit Objectives

At the end of this unit, students will have had opportunities to develop and demonstrate individual development of the following skills:

- Badminton serve
- Underhand clear
- Overhead clear
- Block
- Smash
- Drive

At the end of this unit, students will have had opportunities to develop and demonstrate knowledge and understanding of the following concepts:

- The trajectory that an object takes depends largely on the angle of the racket head on contact and the amount of force generated by the swing.

- All net games include several basic strategies: Always be in a good balanced ready position. Try to send the object to the most open area so that opponents must move to play it. Vary shots so that opponents will have difficulty anticipating what you will do. After every shot, return to the area on the court that gives the best defensive coverage. If working with a partner or a team, communicate with teammates and share coverage of the area.

- Quality competition involves giving 100 percent effort toward the goal of winning but not letting winning become more important than the people involved in the game.

Assessment

The method of formative assessment used during this unit includes Fly, Birdie, Fly—Processing Partner Statements (form 11.1) and Fly, Birdie, Fly—Personal Best Skill Tracking (form 11.2). In addition, Fly, Birdie, Fly—Daily Checkout (form 11.3) is used as a self-assessment of daily class performance. Fly, Birdie, Fly—Peer Assessment (form 11.4) gives students feedback on their use of strategy. The summative assessment used to give students opportunities to demonstrate knowledge and understanding of the strategic use of specific skills is Fly, Birdie, Fly—Strategize! (form 11.5). Although students work on other skills and knowledge during the unit, the primary focus for assessment purposes is on the serve, underhand and overhead clears, and strategy. To avoid surprises, give students this information at the beginning of the unit.

Learning Plan

The following lesson progression was designed to help students meet the goals and objectives identified for this unit, successfully complete the targeted assessments, and have a safe, enjoyable, and educational physical experience.

CONCEPT FOCUS

Angle

SKILL FOCUS

Underhand striking

EQUIPMENT AND MATERIALS

One Fly, Birdie, Fly—Daily Checkout (form 11.3) self-assessment sheet per student; one pencil per student; whiteboard or chart paper; markers; one badminton racket per student; one modified racket or short-handled paddle per student; one or two birdies per student; steel band or Caribbean music; CD player

TEACHING AND LEARNING ACTIVITIES

Setup

The badminton rackets, shorter modified rackets, or paddles suitable for hitting birdies along with badminton birdies should be ready on the sidelines. Before giving equipment to students, discuss how to use rackets safely in the playing area.

Warm-Up—You Choose (5 Minutes)

You can use the warm-up activity called You Choose each time you introduce a new skill or piece of equipment. You Choose gives students a chance to be creative and try different tricks and skills that you may not have thought of. When you give students some freedom, they often come up with wonderful new ideas to incorporate in future lessons. This activity also gives you an opportunity to do a quick general skill assessment before getting started.

Rules and Procedures

1. Students must use equipment safely in self-space.
2. If equipment goes out of a student's space he or she may retrieve it but must return to his or her space before continuing.
3. On the signal to stop, everyone should put his or her equipment on the ground and listen for the next set of instructions.

   Note: Sometimes we forget that middle school students enjoy creative activity as much as elementary school students do. This is an excellent time for students to experiment with the different types of rackets available. Instruct them to choose the racket that they can be most consistent with.

Self-Space Challenge (5 to 8 Minutes)

Self-Space Challenge inspires students to try different tricks with the racket and birdie. They continue to work in self-space. Try to have several birdies available for each student. That way, if a birdie goes out of self-space, the student can use another one without having to move into another person's space.

Directions

1. Begin by telling students that those who were having success striking the birdie during the last activity were using the same type of grip. Ask students if anyone knows what that grip might be (grip as if you were shaking hands with the racket, shake-hands grip). Explain that the grip doesn't change during play. Instead, they change the racket angle with a twisting motion of the shoulder, forearm, and wrist. During this activity have students check their grips often to make sure that they are not letting the racket slip in their hands.

2. Lead them through a series of underhand challenges. The possibilities are limitless. Here are a few to start with:

   - How many times in a row can you hit an underhand forehand shot and stay in self-space?

   - How many times in a row can you hit an underhand backhand shot and stay in self-space?

   - How many times in a row can you alternate between underhand forehand and underhand backhand without letting the birdie land on the ground?

   - Can you strike the birdie, do a 360-degree spin, and hit it again before it hits the ground?

   - Can you strike the birdie in front of you and then, with your racket behind your back, strike it again before it hits the ground?

   - Can you make up striking tricks using the racket and birdie? (Usually with this one you will get a between-the-legs hit. Mention interesting tricks for others to try.)

One on One (8 to 10 Minutes)

After you teach it, you can use One on One, a skill practice activity, with a variety of skills.

Directions

1. On the signal to go, each student faces another person with his or her racket and a birdie. Together they say, "One, two, ready, go . . ." On "Go," both students begin striking the birdie to themselves continuously, attempting to keep it in the air.

2. They continue until one birdie hits the floor. When that happens they shake hands and say, "Good game." The student who was able to perform the skill longer wins that round.

3. Both students move to a designated area (possibly the center circle) to find a new partner to challenge.

4. Students may not turn down a challenge.

Skill Quota (8 to 10 Minutes)

Skill Quota is another activity that you can teach once and then use to practice a variety of skills.

Directions

1. During Skill Quota students begin with a partner and must cooperate to meet a quota that you set to score points.

2. Each time a partnership meets a quota, each person receives 10 points to add to his or her personal score. Then they both move to a designated area to get a new partner and attempt to meet the quota again. You can change the quota or skill any time during the activity.

3. During this game, the skill is partner underhand striking and the quota starts at six hits in a row.

4. One of the partners must catch the sixth hit for the sequence to count.

5. You can challenge students to reach a certain number of points within a designated period.

6. As students participate in this activity, move around the gym giving feedback. Focus on grip and mechanics for underhand striking.

7. After about 10 minutes of play have students sit down with their current partners and listen to the next set of directions.

Two on Two (5 to 8 Minutes)

This activity is played the same way as One on One is played, only the skill is now underhand striking back and forth with a partner. Partnerships travel together and challenge other partnerships to see who can keep the birdies in the air longer.

Closure (3 to 5 Minutes)

At this point gather all students in a circle and give them an overview of the unit, being sure to let them know that they will be involved in cooperative as well as competitive activities throughout the unit. At this time, share the unit objectives. On chart paper or a whiteboard write the following headings: Doing quality work, Being a respectful and responsible class member, Using time efficiently. Ask students to think of what each of those things will look like during the badminton unit. Ask them to use positive terms for each item. For example instead of saying, "Don't mistreat equipment," they might say, "Take care of all equipment." Write their ideas under each heading and let them know that this criterion will be placed on the blank checkout sheet for them to use as a self-assessment at the end of each class period. You can then record the criteria on a blank template and make copies for each student before the next class meeting. Place all copies in a folder marked with the class name and have that available at the end of each class period for student use. After closure at each lesson, students should get their sheets, make their self-assessment, and place the sheet back in the folder. Chapter 2 has more information on using the checkout system for daily assessment.

Lesson #2   Good Serves

CONCEPT FOCUS

Angle of impact, rebound

SKILL FOCUS

Underhand striking, overhead striking, drive smash, block

EQUIPMENT AND MATERIALS

Folder of Fly, Birdie, Fly—Daily Checkout (form 11.3) self-assessment sheets; one pencil per student; one Fly, Birdie, Fly—Personal Best Skill Tracking (form 11.2) sheet per student; whiteboard or chart paper; markers; one badminton racket per student; one modified racket or short-handled paddle per student; three or four birdies per student; nets and net standards (enough to make one court for every four students); court boundary markers for each court; steel band or Caribbean music; CD player

TEACHING AND LEARNING ACTIVITIES

Setup

For the remainder of the unit, you will need to have enough nets to accommodate the number of students that you have in the class. One court for every four students works well. The courts do not have to be standard dimensions for badminton. Remember that the focus here is on the skill and concepts. Although playing on a regulation court would be ideal, it's often not possible. Lack of equipment need not be a barrier. You can construct nets and standards from many different materials. By thinking creatively we can find ways to make things work.

Warm-Up: Fly, Birdie, Fly—Personal Best Skill Tracking (Form 11.2) (8 to 10 Minutes)

This ongoing assessment allows students to work at their own pace. During the entire unit, students can begin the class period with this activity as they enter the gym. The Fly, Birdie, Fly—Personal Best Skill Tracking (form 11.2) assessment template is designed so that several different individual or partner skills can be placed on one sheet. They don't all have to be from the same unit, and you can revisit them throughout the year. The skills that have been added to the template for this unit are self-space underhand hits, partner underhand clears, and serves. Students all have their own score sheets. As students beat their personal best scores, they write in the respective numbers. Students don't have to stop and write in a number each time they beat their score. To maximize activity time, they can keep a mental note of their high score until the end of the designated period and then write it in.

Directions

1. Tell students that each day when they enter the gym, they will get their Fly, Birdie, Fly—Personal Best Skill Tracking sheet and place it and a pencil in a designated area. On some days you will tell them on which skill they are to work. On other days they will have a choice.

2. Begin this introductory lesson by having students hit to themselves. Then assign partners and have them set a score for partner underhand hits.

Good Serves (20 to 25 Minutes)

This serving skill practice activity is always a big hit. The activity is high energy, and games go quickly. You will need to set up courts with boundary lines. Begin with four or five players on each side of a court facing another group of four or five players. In the modified game of badminton used in this unit, any serve landing in bounds is a good serve. The focus is on mechanics and placement.

Directions

1. Teach the basics of the underhand serve with a demonstration and then have students practice their serves by attempting to perform five good serves in a row.

2. After a few minutes of observing and giving positive, specific instructional feedback, stop the action and explain the activity.

3. Tell students that during this game everyone (on both sides of the net) will begin attempting to make good serves.

4. If the birdie lands in bounds, the serve is good and that player continues to serve.

5. If a player's serve lands out of bounds or does not cross the net, he or she must move to the other side of the net and sit in an open space.

6. For that player to return to the business of serving, one of his or her teammates must serve a birdie close enough to the player that he or she can catch it without moving from his or her space on the opposite side of the net.

7. A seated player who catches a birdie may get up and move back with his or her team and start serving again.

8. If all players on one team end up seated before the period ends, the opposing team wins that round. All players return to their original positions, and they play another round.

9. Action is fast, and students have a great time focusing on serve placement. You rotate among groups and give feedback on mechanics.

Closure (3 to 5 Minutes)

Begin by having processing partners stand and face each other somewhere in an open space. Instruct them to sit down when they have come to consensus on how to finish the following statement: "Trajectory is . . ." After a few minutes, as students are beginning to sit down, ask volunteers to share their answers. Use the same procedure for the following partner question: "Two things that will affect trajectory are . . ." Take time to discuss each answer, making sure to point out that the angle of the racket plays a big role in trajectory in badminton. Tell students that during the next class they are going to have a chance to experiment with trajectory with their partners. Before students leave the room, have them check out according to their class performance.

Lesson #3   Angles and Rebound

CONCEPT FOCUS

Angle of impact, rebound

SKILL FOCUS

Underhand striking, overhead striking, drive smash, block

EQUIPMENT AND MATERIALS

Class folder of Fly, Birdie, Fly—Daily Checkout (form 11.3) self-assessment sheets; one pencil per student; class folder of Fly, Birdie, Fly—Personal Best Skill Tracking (form 11.2) sheets; whiteboard or chart paper; markers; one badminton racket per student; one modified racket or short-handled paddle per student; three or four birdies per student; nets and net standards (enough to make one court for every four students); court boundary markers for each court; steel band or Caribbean music; CD player

TEACHING AND LEARNING ACTIVITIES

Setup

Rackets and birdies should be available on the sidelines. Set up nets with lines indicating the boundaries for each court.

Warm-Up: Fly, Birdie, Fly–Personal Best Skill Tracking (Form 11.2)

Using past class performance, choose a skill for students to focus on during this activity or ask them to choose the skill or skills that they feel they need to work on.

Experimenting With Rebound (10 to 15 Minutes)

This guided discovery activity will help students build an understanding of racket angle and rebound.

Directions

1. Set up students in partnerships with one partner facing the other, who will be the feeder. Equip each feeder with 10 birdies.

2. The feeder will practice the serving or underhand clear motion by hitting a birdie to his or her partner across the net.

3. The hitter (partner facing the feeder) should experiment with changing the angle of the racket while making contact with the birdie in an attempt to change the trajectory of the birdie.

4. After the feeder feeds 10 birdies to the hitter, partners change roles. Partners should continue this process until you signal them to stop.

Name the Shots (3 to 5 Minutes)

The names of badminton shots are relatively straightforward, but students always enjoy a guessing game.

Directions

1. Have students place the equipment on the ground and face each other. Tell them that as you watched them experiment, you noticed that most students performed most of the standard badminton shots.

2. Give students three minutes to see if they can come up with the names of those shots.

3. After a few minutes, call on volunteers and lead them to name all the shots while asking them to show you the racket angle for each one.

Coop-Comp (20 to 25 Minutes)

During this cooperative and competitive skill-building activity you can either leave students with their current partners or place them with different partners. They will be experimenting with different shots as in the last activity but in a more dynamic way.

Directions

1. Partners begin by facing each other across the net. When the music starts they need to cooperate by sending the birdie back and forth using friendly underhand clears only. They can see how many times they can successfully hit back and forth without letting the birdie hit the ground.

2. When the music stops, the game changes from a cooperative activity into a competitive challenge. Each partner then attempts to score by using different badminton shots to make the birdie land in his or her partner's court. If space is insufficient to allow partnerships to play this game, have students play doubles style, with two people on each side of the net.

3. Students have a blast trying to anticipate when the music will end. If the music has not resumed and someone scores, the players continue with the competitive mode of this activity until the music starts again. After a few rounds, rotate partners so that students get a chance to work with and compete against others.

Closure (3 to 5 Minutes)

Call students into a circle and ask them to face their processing partners. Hold a racket at a particular angle and ask students to name the shot represented by the angle. They may raise their hands when they come to consensus on the answer. Before students leave the room, have them check out according to their class performance.

CONCEPT FOCUS

Strategy for net games

SKILL FOCUS

Badminton serve, block, underhand clear, overhead clear, smash, drive

EQUIPMENT AND MATERIALS

Class folder of Fly, Birdie, Fly—Daily Checkout (form 11.3) self-assessment sheets; one pencil per student; class folder of Fly, Birdie, Fly—Personal Best Skill Tracking (form 11.2) sheets; whiteboard or chart paper; markers; one badminton racket per student; one modified racket or short-handled paddle per student; three or four birdies per student; nets and net standards (enough to make one court for every four students); court boundary markers for each court; steel band or Caribbean music; CD player

TEACHING AND LEARNING ACTIVITIES

Setup

Have rackets and birdies available on the sidelines. Set up nets with lines or markers indicating the boundaries for each court.

Warm-Up (8 to 10 Minutes): Fly, Birdie, Fly–Personal Best Skill Tracking (Form 11.2)

Using past class performance, choose a skill for students to focus on during this activity or ask them to choose the skill or skills that they feel they need to work on.

Coop–Comp Best of Three (10 to 15 Minutes)

This activity is similar to the Coop–Comp activity in lesson #3, but it introduces scoring.

Directions

1. Set up teams of two (doubles) on the courts available. Have students play the game from the last lesson with the added twist that they will be cooperating while the music is on and then playing a competitive game to 3 points when the music stops.

2. When one team scores 3 points, the teams may start a new game if the music has not yet started.

3. When the music starts again, all groups go back to cooperating.

Top Birds

In this competitive activity you can focus on teaching the strategies for net games. Stop the activity at various intervals and introduce strategies for net games one at a time, having students focus on the new strategy along with the previous one when they begin again. When introducing the strategies ask leading questions and focus on what you notice some students already doing.

Focus on these strategies for net games during this unit:

1. Always maintain an athletic ready position and focus on the play.

2. Send the birdie to the most open area so that your opponent has to move to play it.

3. Use a variety of shots to reduce your opponent's ability to predict what you are going to do from one play to the next.

4. Cover space efficiently by always being in the position that gives you the best coverage.

5. Communicate with your teammate.

Directions

1. Organize students into partnerships or, if you have enough space, have students play singles.

2. If playing with five courts, five partnerships begin on one side of the gym and are designated as top birds. Place challengers across the nets from the top birds. Designate a space as a challenge line where students go when rotating out of the game.

Rules and Directions for Top Birds

1. The serve starts with the top birds. Competitive play does not begin until the birdie has passed over the net twice. In other words, the top birds serve the birdie, and the challengers must return it for play to start. No point can be scored if the serve or return is not good. After the birdie is returned, competitive play begins.

2. After the first point is scored, the team that is ahead serves the birdie. This gives the advantage to the team that is behind.

3. The first team to score 2 points wins the round. If the top birds win the round, they stay where they are and the challengers rotate out of the game to the challenge line. If the challengers win the round, they move under the net to become the top birds. The former top birds rotate out of the game to the challenge line.

4. As courts become available the partnerships in the challenge line move into the challenger spots.

Closure—Team Setup (3 to 5 Minutes)

During the rest of the unit, students work with permanent partners. You can use various methods to set up the partnerships. Your choice will depend on the makeup of the class. An interesting way to assign partners is the random approach of putting names in a hat and drawing out two at a time. Regardless of how you choose to do it, you need to set up partnerships that you can use for the remainder of the unit. After partners are established, have students sit with their new partners and come to consensus on how to complete the following statement: "Two strategies that I will implement for offensive advantage in badminton are . . ." (hit to the open spaces, use a variety of shots, make my opponent move). Discuss their answers. Before students leave the room, have them complete their checkout sheets according to their class performance.

Lesson #5   Teaming Up

CONCEPT FOCUS

Strategy for net games

SKILL FOCUS

Badminton serve, block, underhand clear, overhead clear, smash, drive

EQUIPMENT AND MATERIALS

Class folder of Fly, Birdie, Fly—Daily Checkout (form 11.3) self-assessment sheets; one pencil per student; class folder of Fly, Birdie, Fly—Personal Best Skill Tracking (form 11.2) sheets; whiteboard or chart paper; markers; one badminton racket per student; one modified racket or short-handled paddle per student; three or four birdies per student; nets and net standards (enough to make one court for every four students); court boundary markers for each court; steel band or Caribbean music; CD player; masking tape; a board or poster with the numbers for the ladder tournament written in; one index card for every two students; crayons or colored pencils

TEACHING AND LEARNING ACTIVITIES

Setup

Rackets and birdies should be available on the sidelines. Set up nets with lines or markers indicating the boundaries for each court.

Warm-Up: Fly, Birdie, Fly—Personal Best Skill Tracking (Form 11.2) (8 to 10 Minutes)

Using past class performance, choose a skill for students to focus on during this activity or ask them to choose the skill or skills that they feel they need to work on.

   Note: During the rest of the class period, students will have a chance to begin developing relationships with their partners. You will revisit two activities that students are already familiar with. Throughout the lesson, stop play at various intervals and give instruction on mechanics and strategy for net games as needed. Recognize students who are successfully putting their skills, knowledge, and understanding into action.

Coop–Comp (12 to 15 Minutes)

See lesson #4.

Top Birds (12 to 15 Minutes)

This time the game is played with the teams made in the lesson #4 closure.

Closure (2 to 3 Minutes)

Give each partnership an index card and ask them to decorate it with their names and a team name for the ladder tournament that will begin during the next class period. Put the index cards in a hat or bag so that the students can't see them. Hold the bag up and draw the cards out one by one, placing the cards on the ladder with masking tape, starting with the bottom rung of the ladder. Before students leave the room, have them check out according to their class performance.

The lesson description that follows is for a class tournament. The tournament will take more than one lesson, but the procedure is the same for all three. You may want to use three lessons, but it is possible to use more.

CONCEPT FOCUS

Strategy for net games, racket angle, trajectory

SKILL FOCUS

Badminton serve, block, underhand clear, overhead clear, smash, drive

EQUIPMENT AND MATERIALS

Class folder of Fly, Birdie, Fly—Daily Checkout self-assessment sheets (form 11.3); one pencil per student; class folder of Fly, Birdie, Fly—Personal Best Skill Tracking (form 11.2) sheets; whiteboard or chart paper; markers; one badminton racket per student; one modified racket or short-handled paddle per student; three or four birdies per student; nets and net standards (enough to make one court for every four students); court boundary markers for each court; steel band or Caribbean music; CD player; ladder tournament board designed during the last period; one penny for each court

TEACHING AND LEARNING ACTIVITIES

Setup

Have rackets and birdies available on the sidelines. Set up nets with lines or markers indicating the boundaries for each court.

Warm-Up: Fly, Birdie, Fly–Personal Best Skill Tracking (Form 11.2)

Using past class performance, choose a skill for students to focus on during this activity or ask them to choose the skill or skills that they feel they need to work on.

Ladder Tournament Play (Entire Class Period)

The following procedure for the (modified) ladder tournament works well with the time typically allotted and the need to keep everyone engaged for maximum skill development. The ladder board is already set up from last class, so after the warm-up, have students gather in a circle with their partners. Go over the following rules and procedures.

1. At the beginning of each period, students start by challenging a different team on the ladder.

2. No challenge may be turned down, and no team may play the same team twice in one class period unless a tie game occurs.

3. All games are eight minutes long. Playing for a designated period works better than playing to a certain number of points because kids won't have to wait for long games to end. This way all games end at the same time, allowing for more challenges during the class period.

4. Before each game, teams flip a penny for the serve. All games begin at the same time, and the team that is ahead at the end of the period takes the top space of the two on the ladder. For example, if the team on the sixth rung is ahead of the team on the third rung when time stops,

those teams would switch places on the ladder. If the score is tied at the end of the period, the two teams playing remain on that court and play again during the next period.

5. All teams call their own games and follow the etiquette for net games. Each team calls the lines on their side of the court with no argument from the other team. If a team is unsure of the call they must rule in favor of their opponent. If a major conflict occurs the two teams must meet and come to consensus on how to solve the problem using the established conflict resolution process (see chapter 1). At the end of each game, teams meet at the net, shake hands, and say, "Good game."

6. During the few minutes between games, teams should discuss changes they would like to make in strategy. Then they need to challenge another team.

Thread—At this point you should talk a bit about quality competition and ask questions. Quality competition is competition in which all players play their hardest in an attempt to win the game but also practice respectful behavior toward their opponents during and after the game. Sometimes competitive students fail to remember that the people playing the game are much more important than the game itself. Take time at this point in the tournament to set up students for success by making sure that they understand the expectations surrounding competitive game play. They will have to practice common net game etiquette and will be expected to act as player–referees.

Opponent Strategy Assessment

During lesson #7 or #8, before you begin the tournament, hand out a Fly, Birdie, Fly—Peer Assessment (form 11.4) sheet to each team and instruct them to pay attention to each item as they play their first game of the day. Tell them that they will be filling out this assessment on the team that they play first today. After the first game have students fill out the template and share it with their opponents before they play again. After students review their assessments they should develop a plan to make changes and improve their play for the following games. Giving this assessment early in the tournament allows students to make improvements. An option is to have students do another assessment after their last game and compare the two.

Thread—Whenever students perform peer assessments, you should go over what being objective means and how important it is to be able to set aside personal bias and focus only on the performance.

Closure

For a closure for each of these three classes, have teammates come to consensus on how to complete any combination of the statements on the Fly, Birdie, Fly—Processing Partner Statements (form 11.1). Choose questions based on what you observe during game play. Having that sheet on a clipboard will make it easy to refer to at the end of class. Before students leave the room at the end of each class period, have them complete their checkout sheets according to their class performance.

CONCEPT FOCUS

Strategy for net games

SKILL FOCUS

All badminton skills

EQUIPMENT AND MATERIALS

Class folder of Fly, Birdie, Fly—Daily Checkout (form 11.3) self-assessment sheets; one pencil per student; class folder of Fly, Birdie, Fly—Personal Best Skill Tracking (form 11.2) sheets; one Fly, Birdie, Fly—Strategize! (form 11.5) assessment sheet per student; whiteboard or chart paper; markers; clipboards; one badminton racket per student; one modified racket or short-handled paddle per student; one or two birdies per student; nets and net standards (enough to make one court for every four students); court boundary markers for each court; steel band or Caribbean music; CD player

TEACHING AND LEARNING ACTIVITIES

Setup

In the gym, set up the centers described in the following sections so that as students finish their written assessments they can choose what they would like to do. Give students the written assessment Fly, Birdie, Fly—Strategize! (form 11.5) and go over any questions that they might have. Ask them to complete the form before choosing a center to work at.

Fly, Birdie, Fly–Strategize! (Form 11.5) Written Assessment

Arrange students so that they have space to work on their assessments. Clipboards, pencils, and paper will be needed. As students finish they may move to another center.

Top Bird–One on One

For most of the unit, students have been working with a teammate, and they enjoy having a chance to test their skills on their own. You will need to designate one or two courts as a space for students to play Top Bird. See lesson #4 for directions.

Fly, Birdie, Fly–Personal Best Skill Tracking (Form 11.2)

Some students will want to see if they can top their personal best. You will need to designate one court as a space for them to do that.

Create a Game

Students always have their own ideas on what the rules should be, so why not let them try it? You can use one or two courts for students to use the skills that they gained during the unit to create a new game. Remind them that they need to include everyone interested in participating and that they must use the consensus decision-making process to create the new game. The game must use the skills worked on during the unit.

Primer

If possible you should prime students with what is going to be coming up next. Of course, doing this will depend heavily on what the activity is and how much space is needed. If space is available, you can set out some of the equipment that will be used during the next unit for students to experiment with.

Closure

Gather students together at the end of class and congratulate them on a job well done. Ask them to point out what made the tournament successful and what they might change if they were to do this again. Go over the results on the ladder. Prizes aren't necessary. Students will gain sufficient reward by knowing that they did a good job or by seeing their names on or near the top of the ladder.

Note: Correct the written assessments after class. Hand them back during the next physical education class and go over possible answers. If a student has a question about the scoring of his or her paper, schedule a time to talk about it.

Fly, Birdie, Fly—Processing Partner Statements

Trajectory is …

Two things that will affect trajectory are …

For every game or activity there is a …

Different types of games have different …

Strategy means …

I can't really focus on strategy until I have …

Focusing on strategy requires the ability to …

One strategy common to all types of games is …

Two strategies I will implement to gain offensive advantage in net games are …

Three examples of net games are …

Balance and a good ready position are important in net games because …

Two offensive strategies that I can use to increase my success in net games are …

Two defensive strategies that I can use to increase my success in net games are …

Sending the ball or object to the most open area involves …

The area that will provide me with the most coverage is …

A strategy that I can use in net games that will make it difficult for my opponent to anticipate what I'm going to do is …

Communication between teammates in net games is important because …

Teammates can help improve each other's performance by …

From *Physical Education Assessment Toolkit* by Liz Giles-Brown, 2006, Champaign, IL: Human Kinetics.

Fly, Birdie, Fly—Personal Best Skill Tracking

Name _____ **Grade** _____

Directions: For each skill listed you will be tracking your personal best. Begin by successfully performing the skill as many times as you can while maintaining balance and control. As you work you will be trying to beat your own personal best record. Record a new number only if you beat your previous personal best for each skill.

1. Underhand hits in self-space—badminton

2. Partner underhand clears—badminton

3. Badminton serves

4. _____

5. _____

6. _____

7. _____

8. _____

9. _____

10. _____

Fly, Birdie, Fly—Daily Checkout

Name _____ **Unit** ____ **Badminton**

Directions: Shade in the number that represents each skill if you feel that you met the standard for performance. Be sure that you are practicing honesty when you shade in each number. You may be asked to explain your choices.

1	2	3
1	2	3
1	2	3
1	2	3
1	2	3
1	2	3
1	2	3
1	2	3
1	2	3
1	2	3
1	2	3
1	2	3
1	2	3
1	2	3
1	2	3
1	2	3
1	2	3
1	2	3
1	2	3
1	2	3
1	2	3
1	2	3
1	2	3
1	2	3

1. Doing quality work

- _____
- _____
- _____

2. Being a respectful and responsible classmate

- _____
- _____
- _____

3. Using time efficiently

- _____
- _____
- _____

Fly, Birdie, Fly—Peer Assessment

Performer's Name _____ **Assessor's Name** _____

Directions: Assess your opponent or opponents by shading in the learning line following each strategy that he or she or they use during net activities.

   1. My opponent or opponents maintain an athletic ready position and are focused on the play. It is difficult for me to score.

      never   some of the time   a lot of the time   most of the time

   2. My opponent or opponents attempt to send the ball or object to the most open areas so that I have to move to play it.

      never   some of the time   a lot of the time   most of the time

   3. My opponent or opponents use a variety of shots so that it is hard for me to predict what he or she or they are going to do from one play to the next.

      never   some of the time   a lot of the time   most of the time

   4. My opponent or opponents are always covering space efficiently by consistently being in the position that gives him or her or them the best coverage.

      never   some of the time   a lot of the time   most of the time

Fly, Birdie, Fly—Strategize!

Name _____ **Date** _____

Directions: Describe a situation in which the best strategy would be to use each of the skills in the following list.

1. Underhand clear _____

_____

2. Smash _____

_____

3. Drive _____

_____

4. Block _____

_____

Assessment: Your work will be scored according to the criteria in the following rubric. Use this information to self-assess your work before you hand it in.

4	Excellent work! You went above and beyond!	For each skill listed, the response includes a specific description of a game situation in which the best strategy would be to use that skill. Artwork, specific examples, or details that support answers are included.
3	Good work. Everything is here!	For each skill listed, the response includes a specific description of a game situation in which the best strategy would be to use that skill.
2	Good attempt. Just a few things are missing. Would you like to give it another try?	For at least three of the skills listed, the response includes a specific description of a game situation in which the best strategy would be to use that skill.
1	Let's be sure that you understand. I recommend that you try this one again. See me for more explanation.	For fewer than three of the skills listed, the response includes a specific description of a game situation in which the best strategy would be to use that skill.

From *Physical Education Assessment Toolkit* by Liz Giles-Brown, 2006, Champaign, IL: Human Kinetics.

12

CHAPTER

Planning on Fitness

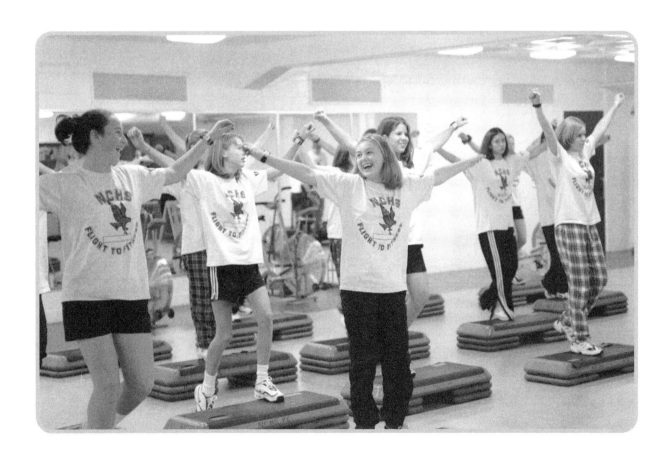

This unit was designed for students in grades five through eight. During this unit, students will be involved in lessons that will teach the various components of health- and skill-related fitness. The unit begins with an introduction to the terms and progresses with activities in which students apply the components of both health- and skill-related fitness to various physical activities. Students get a chance to break down activities into their components and design exercises or drills targeted at improving performance. This unit offers an excellent opportunity to emphasize that people must choose to include fitness as part of their daily lives. In physical education, students will be involved in activities that will have a positive effect on their fitness, but they won't be in physical education classes forever. Ultimately, they will have to decide whether they want to make fitness a habit.

Unit Objectives

At the end of this unit, students will have had opportunities to develop and demonstrate individual development of the following skills:

- Various locomotor movements that they can use in different methods of physical training

- Various axial movements that can be used in different methods of physical training

At the end of this unit, students will have had opportunities to develop and demonstrate knowledge and understanding of the following concepts:

- The components of health-related fitness are cardiorespiratory fitness, flexibility, muscular endurance, muscular strength, and body composition.

- Some of the components of skill-related fitness are coordination, speed, power, agility, balance, and reaction time.

- All physical activities can be broken down into fitness components.

- Personal workouts can be designed with the goal of promoting successful participation in a chosen sport or activity or be designed purely for health-related benefits.

Assessment

The method of formative knowledge and understanding assessment used during this unit includes Planning on Fitness—Thinking About Skill-Related Fitness (form 12.1), a form that contains skill-related fitness knowledge questions that can be copied on the back of Planning on Fitness—Daily Checkout (form 12.2), which is used as a daily class performance self-assessment, and Planning on Fitness—Components (form 12.3). Planning on Fitness—Prescribe It (form 12.4) is used as a summative assessment. This assessment requires students to apply their knowledge and understanding to break an activity into its components and prescribe exercises that will promote successful participation.

Note: The following list describes ways in which you could change certain aspects of this unit to gain flexibility.

- Heart rate measurement—Students use the carotid artery to take their pulse so that they can measure heart rate. If heart rate monitors, watches, or pulse handles are available, students could use those instead.

- Definitions—The specific definitions used for health-related fitness components (cardiorespiratory endurance, flexibility, muscular strength, muscular endurance) and skill-related fitness components (speed, power, balance, agility, coordination, and reaction time) have been left up to you. Many physical educators have found success with specific wordings for definitions, so you must choose your own.

- Target heart rate formula—When target heart rate is used, no absolute value is provided because you may be using this unit with students of various ages. You must choose an appropriate formula or a chart to use with the age level of your students.

Learning Plan

The following lesson progression was designed to help students meet the goals and objectives identified for this unit, successfully complete the targeted assessments, and have a safe, enjoyable, and educational physical experience.

Lesson #1 Introductions

CONCEPT FOCUS

Health- and skill-related fitness vocabulary, cardiorespiratory fitness

SKILL FOCUS

Measuring heart rate

EQUIPMENT AND MATERIALS

One card each with the following terms: cardiorespiratory endurance, flexibility, muscular strength, muscular endurance, body composition, power, speed, balance, reaction time, agility, and coordination; one card each with the definition that you choose to use for each of the fitness terms; one piece of paper per student; one pencil per student; CD player and music; stopwatch; one copy of Planning on Fitness—Thinking About Skill-Related Fitness (form 12.1) copied on the reverse side of Planning on Fitness—Daily Checkout (form 12.2)

TEACHING AND LEARNING ACTIVITIES

Setup

Have blank papers and pencils available in one area on the perimeter of the activity area for students to use throughout the lesson. Have one copy of Planning on Fitness—Thinking About Skill-Related Fitness (form 12.1) copied on the reverse side of Planning on Fitness—Daily Checkout (form 12.2) in a folder for class use throughout the unit available for the end of class (referred to as the checkout folder from here on).

Warm-Up and Introduction (10 to 15 Minutes)

As students enter the gym, hand each one a card with either a term or a definition on it. You'll need 22 cards: 11 with terms and 11 with definitions. If you have more than 22 students in the class, have a few students double up on one card.

Directions

1. Ask each student to find an open space, read his or her card, and listen to the directions. Tell them that each card has a match that someone else is holding. If they have a word or term, then the match will be the definition and vice versa. Their job is to find the person who has the match as quickly as they can. Tell them that you will be timing the entire class.

2. When they find a match they should sit down. You will check to see whether they are correct. If they are not correct you will ask them to get up and try again. If they are correct they stay seated and do flexibility or muscular endurance routines while waiting for their classmates to find their matches (see chapter 1 for more information about fitness routines). On your signal to begin finding matches, you start the stopwatch.

3. When all students have found their correct matches, call them into a circle, give them their time for the activity, and have each student read a term and definition. Talk briefly about how all physical activities and skills are made up of parts called components and that they are going to learn about each component. By having this knowledge they will be able to look at skills and activities and break them down into their health- and skill-related parts. Tell them that throughout the unit they will be developing the knowledge and skills necessary to put together health- and skill-related workouts that will help them reach specific health and performance goals.

4. Collect the cards and let students know that later in the unit they will have opportunities to beat their original score.

5. Give each student a copy of Planning on Fitness—Thinking About Skill-Related Fitness (form 12.1), copied on the reverse side of Planning on Fitness—Daily Checkout (form 12.2). Explain that at the end of class they will be checking out according to the class criteria, when they will also have opportunities to complete parts of Planning on Fitness—Thinking About Skill-Related Fitness. Be sure they understand that they can answer the questions at their own pace but that they must finish by the last class period.

Thread—Developing fitness routines that students can use at any time promotes efficient use of time in physical education classes. See chapter 1 for more information on developing fitness routines.

Focus on Cardiorespiratory Fitness (10 to 15 Minutes)

This guided discovery activity will help students build an understanding of how heart rate relates to intensity in cardiorespiratory activities.

Directions

1. As you move around the circle and collect the cards, ask students to move to the area where you have the blank papers and pencils. Students should put their names on the top of their papers.

2. After they have done that, instruct them to find their pulse rate by placing their index and middle fingers on the carotid artery. Have students raise the opposite hand when they have located their pulse so that you know who might need help.

3. After all students have been able to locate their pulse, have them move to an open space. Tell them that during the next activity they will be participating in activities of different intensity. They will need to find their pulse, start counting on the signal to start, and stop counting on the signal to stop. Each time they need to count, you direct them to the papers, give the signal to start and stop the count, and then give the next set of instructions. They will be counting for 15 seconds.

4. When all students are ready, instruct them to pretend that they have gone to the mall for the afternoon with some friends and are just strolling along doing some window shopping, occasionally stopping to look at something more closely. Tell them that they have the entire afternoon and are not in a hurry. Walk around with them and lead the activity by adding images and situations to make it fun and interesting. For instance, you might say, "Up ahead you notice a sale on fleece sweatshirts that are popular now." Or you could say, "You meet a group of friends and stop to chat for a while and then move on." After a few minutes of this have students move to the papers, remain standing, and be ready to count. Time them for 15 seconds and then signal them to stop. Ask them to write the word *mall* on their papers and the number that they counted when they took their pulse.

5. You will use this process for each of the following scenarios. Each one should take two or three minutes. Each time, have students move to the papers, remain standing, count, and record. Give them a word for each recording.

Late

Tell students to move through the area as if they were late for a flight that was going to take off in 10 minutes. They are at one end of a large airport, and the plane is at the other. They can't run because the concourse is too crowded, but they can power walk, dodging and weaving in and out of the other people.

Dog Jog

The students have signed on to dog sit for their neighbor's large dog. They were instructed to take the dog for a walk every morning. The dog doesn't quite understand what walk means, so they end up jogging with it for about 20 minutes each day.

Tag Break

Tell students that they have been inside working hard on a state test for about two hours. The teacher knows that they need a break, so he or she takes them to the gym to play a tag game (use one of their favorites). Students are ready for some activity and are excited to be moving.

Closure (2 to 3 Minutes)

Have students take their pulse recordings to an area suited for a closure activity. Assign processing partners for the remainder of the unit. (Processing partners are two students assigned to process information together during specified lessons. Chapter 9 covers this in depth.) Ask students to face their partners and share anything that they noticed about what happened to their heart rate. Take volunteers to answer after partners have shared with each other. Talk for a minute about how heart rate measures the intensity of a cardiorespiratory workout. If they multiplied the number of beats that they counted in 15 seconds by four, they would know how many times their hearts were beating in each minute. Then ask partnerships to come to consensus on the answer to the following statement: "Cardiorespiratory fitness is . . ." (answers might include using the heart and lungs to exercise, being able to last for long periods while working at medium intensity). Take volunteers and briefly discuss answers. Then tell students that they have had some practice taking their pulse so their assignment is to take their pulse for 15 seconds one morning before they get out of bed and bring that number to the next class meeting. Have students fill in their checkout sheets based on their class performance before they leave.

Lesson #2 Cardio and Agility

CONCEPT FOCUS

Cardiorespiratory fitness, target heart rate, agility

SKILL FOCUS

Maintaining the target heart rate intensity, moving at top speed with quick changes in direction

EQUIPMENT AND MATERIALS

Heart rate measurements from the last class, pencils, target heart rate ranges for students, five cones or markers for every two students, class checkout folder, music, CD player

TEACHING AND LEARNING ACTIVITIES

Setup

Have the heart rate measurements out from last class along with a pencil for each student.

Warm-Up (3 to 5 Minutes)

As students enter the gym direct them to their heart rate measurements from the last class. Ask them to write the word *resting* on the paper and to record the resting heart rate that they took before getting out of bed. Explain that the true resting heart rate can be measured only during sleep but that the best we can do is take a measurement before rising in the morning.

After they have recorded their heart rate ask them to begin walking in open spaces to the music until they hear the signal to stop. When you have them stop, ask them to find their pulse and count. They will take their pulse for 15 seconds. After this measurement, ask students the following question: "How do we measure the intensity of a cardiorespiratory workout?" (heart rate). Take volunteers until someone comes up with the correct answer. Tell them that everyone has a target heart rate that he or she can shoot for to give the heart a good workout. A person's target heart rate will depend on his or her age and fitness level. Give them the numbers that you plan to use for their target heart rates and tell them to be ready to move, to listen for the signal to stop, and to be ready to count.

What Does My Target Feel Like? (10 to 15 Minutes)

During this activity, students will participate in an experiment that will help them find out what it feels like to work in their target zone.

Directions

1. Give them the signal to start walking again. As they walk tell them that they will be increasing their speed slightly during each interval and that it is important that they not increase it too much each time. They are not to increase their speed until you instruct them to.

2. After two or three minutes have students take their pulse for 15 seconds. If they are in their zone tell them to continue to work at that intensity. If they are not working within their zone they should increase their intensity slightly.

3. Follow this procedure until all students are working within their target zones. Stress the fact that people are different and that each person will require a different intensity level to reach his or her target zone.

4. This activity will give students an idea of what it feels like to maintain their target zone intensity for a time. If they work too hard they will not be able to maintain their intensity. Continue until all students are working within their target zones.

5. Ask students to stand facing their processing partners and come to consensus on what the words *duration* and *frequency* mean (duration is how long; frequency is how often). If they are able to come to consensus they should sit down to signal that they are finished. Ask volunteers to answer the question.

6. Tell students that they now know how hard they need to work to get a good cardiorespiratory workout. Now they need to find out how often and how long they need to work. Ask students to come to consensus on how often a person should participate in cardiorespiratory activities (at least three times per week) and how long they should work when they do (at least 20 minutes). Take answers and briefly discuss how much time that takes out of a person's schedule.

Agility (10 to 15 Minutes)

Before starting this portion of the lesson, organize students with new partners.

Thread—Before giving the signal, remind students about how they communicate with body language and to practice the virtue of kindness as they get partners.

Directions

1. As students find their partners, arrange five cones in the pattern illustrated in the following diagram.

2. Ask students if they remember the definition of agility from the first activity of this fitness unit. Have them think back to the activity in which they had to match definitions with health- and skill-related fitness components. Ask volunteers to share until you have a correct answer.

3. Tell students that they are going to participate in an agility drill. Show them how to move through the pattern illustrated in the diagram and then ask them to get five markers, set them up, and practice walking the pattern until you ask them to stop.

4. They can choose to follow each other through the pattern, or they can take turns. Tell them that the idea is to be able to do the drill as fast as they can without missing a cone.

5. After students are familiar with the pattern tell them that they are going to take turns moving through the pattern as quickly as they can for 30 seconds. Each time they pass the start cone they score 1 point. Their objective is to see how many times they can pass the start cone in the 30-second interval. Partners should count for each other.

6. Each student should have two or three attempts to beat his or her original score.

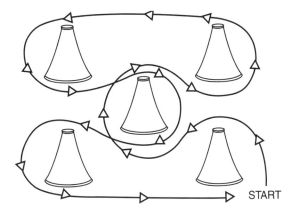

Closure (2 to 3 Minutes)

Ask students to face their processing partners and come up with two activities that require high levels of cardiorespiratory fitness to be successful (basketball, soccer, cross-country skiing, swimming, and so on) and two activities that require high levels of agility to be successful (soccer, basketball, football, tennis, badminton). Ask students to share their answers. Tell them that all activities can be broken down into components of health- and skill-related fitness. When athletes are able to break down their sport into its components, they can train the movements and components that will lead to more success. Have students fill in their checkout sheet according to class performance and answer questions on the reverse side if they are ready.

Lesson #3   More Components

CONCEPT FOCUS

Coordination, balance, power, speed, muscular endurance

SKILL FOCUS

Basketball layup, jumping, jumping rope, running

EQUIPMENT AND MATERIALS

Cards with definitions and components from lesson #1, three or four basketballs, three or four jump ropes, three or four polyspots, three or four balance boards, one stopwatch, one tape measure, two gymnastic mats for curl-ups, four cones, whiteboard or chart paper, markers, class checkout folder

TEACHING AND LEARNING ACTIVITIES

Setup

Set up the gym in station format and divide the students into seven even groups. The following list describes what each station should look like. The instructions are included. When you give the instructions do not disclose what part of fitness each station represents.

1. Layups (coordination)—Have basketballs available for students to practice layup shots.
2. Standing broad jump (power)—Set up a tape measure at a jumping line. Tape it to the floor so that students can measure how far they jump. They take turns, using a two-foot takeoff and two-foot landing.
3. One foot (balance)—Place polyspots on the ground. Students see how long they can balance on one foot while swinging their opposite foot forward and backward. Each student in the group stands on a spot with one foot. On the signal from one student, they see who can last the longest.
4. Curl-ups (muscular endurance)—Place gymnastics mats on the floor. Students see how many curl-ups they can do in a row without stopping.
5. Crossover jump rope trick (coordination)—Place jump ropes in one area. Students practice the crossover move, arms alternately crossing and uncrossing as they jump the rope.
6. Balance or bolo board (balance)—Place balance boards (boards on round tubes) in one area. Students take turns seeing how long they can keep both ends of the board off the ground.
7. Sprints (speed)—Mark a start line and a finish line with cones and have a stopwatch available for timing. On the "Ready, set, go" signal, students time each other in sprints from one end of the room to the other.

Warm-Up (3 to 5 Minutes)

As students enter the door, repeat the activity that they did in lesson #1 with the definitions and components. Tell them that as they move to find partners, they are trying to beat their score from the first day. Also instruct them to avoid any equipment that might be out. As students find matches, move to check whether they are correct. If they are correct, they stay and do a fitness routine (if routines have been established; see chapter 1). If they are incorrect they get up and continue looking for the correct match.

Mystery Stations (20 to 30 Minutes)

Students work at each station for three or four minutes. The purpose of the stations is to have students experience the components represented and be cognitively engaged in trying to figure out what each one is.

Directions

1. After the warm-up activity, organize students into their groups and give them the instructions for each station. Tell them that one station represents a component of health-related fitness and that six stations represent components of skill-related fitness.

2. Tell students that their job is to participate in a station, stop on the signal, and come to consensus with their group members on what health- or skill-related fitness component is represented. They then move to the next station to begin again.

Closure (2 to 3 Minutes)

Ask group members to sit beside each other and gather in one area of the gym. Point to each station and ask students what component their group believes it represents. On a whiteboard or chart paper make a list of the components that were part of the mystery stations and ask students to remember what they did during the last class (cardiorespiratory and agility). Ask the class as a whole to come up with two activities in which high levels of each component are necessary for successful participation. Then ask them if anyone can remember what components are left (muscular strength, flexibility, body composition). Take volunteers and complete the list with their answers. Have students fill in their checkout sheets according to class performance and to answer any questions on the reverse side if they are ready.

Lesson #4   Twofer

CONCEPT FOCUS

Cardiorespiratory endurance, muscular endurance

SKILL FOCUS

Axial movements, locomotor movements

EQUIPMENT AND MATERIALS

A pair of two-pound (one-kilogram) hand weights for every two students, jogging or power-walking space, one carpet square or mat for every two students, one beanbag for every two students, music, CD player, class checkout folder, one copy of Planning on Fitness—Components (form 12.3)

TEACHING AND LEARNING ACTIVITIES

Setup

Set up one carpet square, two small hand weights, and one beanbag for every two students in a large circle in the center of the movement area.

Warm-Up

As students walk into the gym, instruct them to walk briskly around the gym. While they walk, instruct them to stretch and reach in different directions with their arms (forward, up, across, and so on). After a few minutes, as they are still walking, ask pairs of students to move to carpet squares and stand one behind the other.

Twofer (20 Minutes)

During this activity, students will receive a twofer (two for the price of one). They will get both a cardiorespiratory workout and a muscular strength and endurance workout.

Directions

1. Ask the class if anyone knows what a twofer is. Lead them with clues to answer that a twofer is two articles for the price of one. Ask if anyone has ever been lucky enough to be on the receiving end of a twofer. They may answer that they received twofers on CDs, T-shirts, or food items. Tell students that this is their lucky day because they are about to receive a twofer in physical education class. At the end of class, their job will be to figure out what two things they received.

2. Tell students that one partner will either power walk or jog while the other partner does the activity that you will be demonstrating.

3. After one minute you will give them the signal to switch, at which time the partner who was following along with you will begin power walking or jogging and the other partner will come to join the circle and follow along with the stationary activity.

4. Tell them that they will do each activity—the stationary activity and power walking or jogging—eight times for a total of 16 minutes. Their job is to make the transition quickly, stay within their target heart rate zone for the entire activity, and perform slow, controlled movements when they are following what you are doing. The activity ends up taking about 20 minutes including the transitions. The following is a list of activities that you can use with this lesson, although you can use any muscular endurance activity.

   • Punches—Alternately punch forward with the right hand and then the left hand, holding a small hand weight in each hand and holding the extended arm out for a count of one.

   • Triceps—With hand weights held straight overhead, alternately bend the elbows so that the upper arm stays up but the forearm moves down toward the back.

   • Beanbag eights—Sitting on the carpet square, balanced on the buttocks, pass the beanbag around the legs in a figure-eight pattern without letting the heels contact the ground. Pass the beanbag under the left leg with the right hand and pass it to the left hand. Then pass the beanbag with the left hand over the top of the left leg, under the right leg, and into the right hand, which starts the figure-eight pattern again.

   • Arm circles—Do slow, controlled arm circles with hand weights.

   • Biceps—Do biceps curls, alternating between the right arm and the left arm, being sure to hold the upper arms at the sides.

   • Push cross—In the push-up position, alternately touch the opposite shoulder with one hand and then the other.

   • Ceiling press—With hand weights held at shoulder height and elbows bent, press upward to the ceiling, first with one arm and then the other.

   • Front straddles—Keeping weight evenly distributed on both feet, jump and straddle forward, bending the knees on landing to absorb the force. Push upward again and change foot position so that the opposite foot is now forward.

Cool-Down (2 to 3 Minutes)

After they complete all intervals, have students cool down by walking with the music around the outside of the area. Ask them to be thinking about the two things that they just received. When students have cooled down, lead them in some flexibility exercises to stretch their warm muscles. As they perform the flexibility exercises, review the definition of flexibility and its benefits.

Closure (2 to 3 Minutes)

Gather students in one area and ask them to stand facing their processing partners. Ask students to come to consensus on what the twofer was today (cardiorespiratory and muscular endurance) and ask them to share their answers. Then ask students to share with their partners the definitions of the two components and one of their favorite physical activities that requires cardiorespiratory endurance, muscular endurance, or both to be successful. After a minute ask them to raise their hands to share with the rest of the group. Hand each student a copy of Planning on Fitness—Components (form 12.3) and ask them to complete it for homework. Have students fill in their checkout sheet according to class performance and answer any questions on the reverse side if they are ready.

Lesson #5 Through Lesson #7   What's Out There?

CONCEPT FOCUS

Health- and skill-related fitness components

SKILL FOCUS

Breaking down activities into movements and components

EQUIPMENT AND MATERIALS

Equipment based on the guests and activities chosen, class checkout folder

TEACHING AND LEARNING ACTIVITIES

Setup and Warm-Up

The guest and activity will determine setup and warm-up.

Guest Presenters (30 to 35 Minutes)

Most communities have various activity opportunities for adults and kids. YMCAs and youth clubs offer many activities that address the components of health- and skill-related fitness. These three lessons are dedicated to having guest presenters share some of those activities with students in an active way. Students enjoy trying new things and may discover an activity that they want to pursue in the future. Instructors are often willing to come in and share what they do with students. Their job is to introduce an activity and lead the class in a sample workout. Activities can include but are not limited to yoga, Pilates, cardio kickboxing, step aerobics, and various types of aerobic exercise classes. As students participate in the workout they should be thinking about what components of health- and skill-related fitness are targeted by the workout.

Closure (3 to 5 Minutes)

At the end of each class encourage students to ask questions. Then have them stand with their processing partners and come to consensus on what components they worked on during the lesson. They sit down to signal that they are finished. After students are seated ask them to share their answers. Have students fill in their checkout sheet according to class performance and answer any questions on the reverse side if they are ready. Announce that by the end of the seventh class they need to have completed Planning on Fitness—Thinking About Skill-Related Fitness (form 12.1). You should correct these after the seventh class and hand them back at the beginning of the eighth class.

Lesson #8   Break It Down

CONCEPT FOCUS

Health- and skill-related fitness components

SKILL FOCUS

A variety of axial and locomotor movements associated with different sports or physical activities

EQUIPMENT AND MATERIALS

CD or tape player; music; a variety of cones, spots, hoops, mats, and any other equipment that could be used to develop fitness moves for sports or physical activities; class checkout folder

TEACHING AND LEARNING ACTIVITIES

Setup

Place all equipment around the perimeter of the room so that it is available for students to use.

Warm-Up

As students enter the gym, hand them their Planning on Fitness—Thinking About Skill-Related Fitness (form 12.1) sheets and ask them to walk around the perimeter of the gym. As they walk, ask them to read over their answers and any feedback given. Call them in and ask volunteers to answer the questions. If any student has a question about his or her score, arrange to talk with the student individually.

Walk On (5 to 8 Minutes)

Ask students to walk slowly around the room. When the music pauses they are to increase their speed slightly. Eight pauses will occur, so students should increase their pace slowly. At the end of this activity ask students to stand facing their processing partners and come to consensus on the answer to the following question: "If we were to continue this activity for 20 minutes, what part of health-related fitness would you be working to improve?" (cardiorespiratory fitness). Ask volunteers to answer.

Training for Specific Activities (20 to 25 Minutes)

This activity helps students apply their knowledge of health- and skill-related fitness components to come up with training moves for specific activities.

Directions

1. Begin by talking about how athletes who really want to improve performance break down their sport into its components to work on sport-specific training. Remind students that some people have health-related goals, which is great. But when a person wants to excel at a specific sport, he or she can focus on health- and skill-related components at the same time.

2. Place students in groups of three or four and tell them that they are going to be breaking down an activity and designing training moves specific to that activity. Tell them that you are going to name a sport or activity. Their job is to identify one component and one movement specific to the activity. After their group has identified a component and movement, they must come up with a training move that targets both.

3. To make sure that everyone understands the instructions, perform the following demonstration.

   > Pretend that you are a student and that the teacher just said that the activity is volleyball. Role-play your thought process as you complete the task. You might say the following as you act out the role of a student. "Let me see now, I know that blocking is an important skill in volleyball. Blocking involves being able to perform a vertical jump as high as possible after moving forward. Jumping as high as I can one time requires power. So power is the skill-related component that I want to focus on, and jumping is the movement. Hmmm, what pieces of equipment over there could I use to set up a training move? I think I'll just need two spots." Then demonstrate a training move by putting two spots on the floor. Start at one spot and move quickly forward to the other one. When you reach the other spot, jump as high as you can and extend your arms up over your head. Then jog quickly backward to the first spot and repeat the movement. Repeat the movement several times.

4. Let students know that after you name each activity they will have five minutes to identify a component and a movement and then come up with a training activity.

5. After they come up with the training activity, they need to practice it so that their group can demonstrate it for the rest of the class when it is their turn. At this point give students their first sport or activity. Choose one based on what students are interested in.

6. Walk around the room and ask clarifying questions as students work within their groups.

7. When you see that students are finished, ask all students to have a seat. Ask groups to share what they identified as the component and the movement and then show their training move.

8. After they complete the first one, give students another sport or activity. Do as many as time allows during the class period.

Closure (2 to 3 Minutes)

Ask students to sit with their group members and come to consensus on a sport or activity that they would like to use during the next class period. Tell them that they must keep their choice a secret because the rest of the class will be guessing what they chose at some point during the class period. After they come to consensus they need to tell you what their activity will be and mark their checkout sheets based on their class performance.

Lesson #9   Guessing Games

CONCEPT FOCUS

Health- and skill-related fitness components

SKILL FOCUS

A variety of axial and locomotor movements associated with sports or physical activities

EQUIPMENT AND MATERIALS

CD or tape player; music; cones, spots, hoops, mats, and any equipment that could be used to develop fitness moves for sports or physical activities; class checkout folder

TEACHING AND LEARNING ACTIVITIES

Setup

Place all equipment on the perimeter of the room so that it is available for students to use.

Warm-Up (2 to 3 Minutes)

As students enter the gym ask them to gather with their group members from the previous class period. Ask them to stand in a line one behind another so that they are at least an arm's length apart. When the music starts, the lead person starts a slow jog into open spaces. The person at the back of the line chooses any other locomotor movement (gallop, skip, slide, leap, and so on) and performs it at a faster speed to move from the back of the line to the front so that he or she becomes the new leader. When that person reaches the front of the line, he or she begins a slow jog. The person now last in line chooses a locomotor movement and performs it as he or she moves to the front. After a few minutes ask students to stand in a circle in their groups and quietly remind each other what sport or activity they picked yesterday.

Stump the Class (30 to 35 Minutes)

In this activity students use the skills that they developed during the previous class period to create four training moves specific to their chosen activity.

Directions

1. Tell students that they may use any of the equipment available to complete the task.

2. All groups have 20 minutes to design four training moves related to their chosen sport, practice them, and be ready to present to the rest of the class.

3. After each presentation, the rest of the class tries to guess what sport or activity the group was working on based on the movements and components chosen.

4. Take any questions that the groups may have and then walk around giving feedback and troubleshooting.

5. At the time deadline give each group a chance to perform and entertain guesses.

6. If the available time does not permit all groups to perform during one class period, you can extend this lesson to the next class meeting. If that happens, hold on to the assessment sheet until everyone has had a chance to perform.

Closure (3 to 5 Minutes)

Hand out the assessment sheet Planning on Fitness—Prescribe It (form 12.4) and ask students to read the instructions. Tell students that they are going to have an opportunity to show what they have learned by completing this assessment. Using all the work that they have done on skill-related fitness during the unit, they are to choose an activity that was not addressed during the last two class periods, develop two training moves that they could prescribe for the activity, and describe them in the spaces provided. Assign a due date and answer any questions that students might have. Tell students that this will be the last class period in this unit and prime them with the unit that they will be participating in next. Ask them to mark their checkout sheets according to their class performance before they leave. During the first class of the next unit, return all the assessments completed during this unit and go over the answers as a group. After correcting the assessments, return them and have students read any feedback given. If any student has questions about his or her score, arrange to meet one on one.

Planning on Fitness—Thinking About Skill-Related Fitness

Name _____ **Date** _____

Directions: Complete the following statements about skill-related fitness by using the words provided.

1. A _____ movement is smooth and efficient with little wasted motion.

2. When someone is able to change direction quickly when moving at top speed, we say that he or she has a lot of _____.

3. Moving from one place to another in the shortest time possible requires great _____.

4. In a powerful movement, a person uses strong _____ in one explosive act.

5. _____ balance requires a person to maintain equilibrium while still.

6. Dynamic _____ involves maintaining equilibrium while moving.

7. The _____ is a movement that requires power.

8. When playing defense against someone who is able to change _____ quickly, you must be agile.

9. A juggler must have high levels of _____ to keep all those balls in the air.

10. Many physical activities involve different combinations of health-related fitness components and _____-related fitness components.

coordinated	speed	static	direction	agility
force	balance	skill	coordination	standing broad jump

Scoring: The number of correct answers _____ divided by the number of possible answers _____ equals the percentage of correct answers _____.

Planning on Fitness—Daily Checkout

Name _____ **Unit** _____

Directions: Shade in the number that represents each skill if you feel that you met the standard for performance. Be sure that you are practicing honesty when you shade in each number. You may be asked to explain your choices.

I	2	3
I	2	3
I	2	3
I	2	3
I	2	3
I	2	3
I	2	3
I	2	3
I	2	3
I	2	3
I	2	3
I	2	3
I	2	3
I	2	3
I	2	3
I	2	3
I	2	3
I	2	3
I	2	3
I	2	3
I	2	3
I	2	3
I	2	3
I	2	3
I	2	3
I	2	3

1. Doing quality work

- I remained on task and focused on the specific skill cues for today's skill or lesson.
- I worked to improve skills today.
- I persevered by having an "I can" attitude.

2. Being a respectful and responsible classmate

- I listened to my classmates and made eye contact. I didn't interrupt.
- I tried to be creative and open-minded.
- I gave effort, energy, and enthusiasm to the tasks.
- When a decision needed to be made, I didn't give orders. I used the consensus decision-making process.
- If involved in a conflict, I used conflict resolution skills, "I" statements, and a calm, soft voice instead of a loud, angry voice.

3. Using time efficiently

- I carried out directions and transitions quickly and quietly.
- I responded to signals immediately and appropriately.

Planning on Fitness—Components

Name _____ **Date** _____

   1. What are three components of health-related physical fitness? _____

     _____

     _____

     _____

     _____

     _____

   2. What are three components of skill-related fitness? _____

     _____

     _____

     _____

     _____

     _____

Scoring: The number of correct answers _____ divided by the number of possible answers _____ equals the percentage of correct answers _____.

Planning on Fitness—Prescribe It

Name _____ **Date** _____

Directions: Jessie wants to train for _____. Identify two skill-related fitness components that are important for her to develop to be successful in this activity. For each component, prescribe one exercise or activity that she can add to her workout to help reach her training goals.

1._____   2._____

_____   _____

_____   _____

_____   _____

_____   _____

_____   _____

_____   _____

_____   _____

_____   _____

_____   _____

_____   _____

_____   _____

Assessment: Your work will be scored according to the criteria in the following rubric. Use this information to self-assess your work before you hand it in.

4	Excellent work! You went above and beyond!	Each response is complete and correct. Two skill-related fitness components are identified, and a prescription for a related training activity for each is provided. Artwork, specific examples, or details that support answers are included.
3	Good work. Everything is here!	Each response is complete and correct. Two skill-related fitness components are identified, and a prescription for a related training activity for each is provided.
2	Good attempt. Just a few things are missing. Would you like to try this one again?	One item is missing or incorrect. One of the two skill-related fitness components identified or a related exercise or activity is incorrect.
1	Let's be sure that you understand. I recommend that you try this one again. See me for more explanation.	No complete and correct answers are provided. Skill-related fitness components or related training activities are incorrect or missing.

Appendix

ANSWER KEYS AND GUIDELINES

This appendix contains the answers to many of the assessments included in the book and on the accompanying CD-ROM. For the assessments that do not have one correct answer, guidelines are provided for you to use as you review student work. The answers to the assessments are organized by chapter. The name of the assessment follows the form number to facilitate reference.

Chapter 2: Checkout: Daily Self-Assessment System

2.1–2.6 Physical Education Daily Checkout 1-6—The answers to these self-reflection assessments will depend on student performance and the student's ability to make an objective assessment of his or her class performance.

2.7 Thinking About Flexibility—1. stretch, 2. hurt, pain, 3. bouncing, 4. flexibility, 5. long, tight, 6. joints, 7. injured, 8. cold

2.8 Thinking About Cardiorespiratory Fitness—1. time, 2. heart, 3. gradual, 4. carbohydrates, 5. respiratory, oxygen, 6. older, 7. lungs, 8. jogging, 9. three

2.9 Practicing Virtues—Answers will depend on the student's experience during each lesson. Look for specific versus general answers.

2.10 Thinking About Muscular Strength and Muscular Endurance—1. force, 2. tired, 3. posture, 4. health, 5. endurance, 6. strength, 7. burst, 8. legs, 9. upper, 10. more

2.11 Thinking About Skill-Related Fitness—1. coordinated, 2. agility, 3. speed, 4. force, 5. static, 6. balance, 7. standing broad jump, 8. direction, 9. coordination, 10. skill

2.12 Thinking About Fitness Training—1. long, 2. often, 3. hard, 4. more, 5. increasing, 6. heart rate, 7. overload, 8. intensity, 9. muscular endurance, 10. target heart rate

2.13 Thinking About Physiological Changes—1. F, 2. T, 3. T, 4. F, 5. T, 6. T, 7. T, 8. T, 9. F, 10. T

2.14 Physical Education Team Checkout—The answers to these self-reflection assessments will depend on student performance.

2.15 Virtue Clue Cards

1. You practice this virtue when dealing with all people. Sometimes it's hard when you are having a disagreement, but someone who practices this virtue will treat all people with consideration.—Respect

2. People who practice this virtue are willing to accept the consequences for their own actions whether those consequences are bad or good.—Responsibility

3. This virtue is a voice inside your head that says, "If at first you don't succeed, try, try again." This virtue doesn't let you give up.—Perseverance

4. You use this virtue to manage your behavior and help you control yourself. This virtue is the one that tells you to do your homework before you go outside to play.—Self-discipline

5. If you regularly practice this virtue, you are always truthful no matter what, even if it means that you might get into trouble.—Honesty

6. When you practice this virtue, you try to understand how another person feels in certain situations. This ability helps you care for others.—Compassion

7. When you are afraid, you will call on this virtue to do what you know you should do or need to do.—Courage

8. People who possess this virtue are dependable. You can always trust that they will do the right thing.—Trustworthiness

Chapter 3: Setting Goals and Reflecting on Performance

The content of the responses in all assessments in chapter 3 will depend on the unit being taught. General guidelines and examples of what to look for when students set goals and reflect on their performance are provided here.

Goal-Setting Assessments

3.1 Setting Goals for Improvement

3.2 Working to Improve Our Community

3.3 Setting Goals and Reflecting

For assessments 3.1 through 3.3, in which students are asked to set a personal goal, look for specific measurable goals rather than vague answers. For example, "I want to dribble better" or "I want to get better at soccer" would be unacceptable. These goals are not specific or measurable. "I would like to be able to dribble the ball and keep it close to my feet so that it's harder for the defense to steal" would be a more specific, acceptable goal.

Reflection Assessments

3.1 Setting Goals for Improvement

3.2 Working to Improve Our Community

3.3 Setting Goals and Reflecting

3.4 Unit Reflections 1

3.5 Unit Reflections 2

3.6 Reflecting on My Work in Physical Education

For assessments 3.1 through 3.6, in which students are asked to reflect on their performance or their personal goals, look for answers stated in specific terms rather than general terms. For example, to provide evidence of improvement, an acceptable response would have to say more than simply "I did better." An acceptable answer might be "I know I improved my soccer dribbling because at the beginning of the unit people were able to steal the ball easily when I was dribbling. Now I can control the ball longer and it's harder for the defense to steal it."

Reflection Bar Graph or Checklist Assessments

3.4 Unit Reflections 1

3.6 Reflecting on My Work in Physical Education

3.7 Reflections Quick Check

For assessments 3.4, 3.6, and 3.7, in which students are asked to shade in a bar graph based on performance or complete a checklist, the student's response will depend on his or her ability to reflect objectively on his or her performance. If after reviewing a student's assessment you note a significant discrepancy between what you see happening and what the student sees happening, you should provide further instruction on either an individual basis or a group basis, depending on need.

Chapter 4: On the Move With Motor Skills

The content of the responses in all assessments in chapter 4 will depend on the unit that is being taught. General guidelines and examples of what to look for in student responses are provided here.

Skill Cue Assessments

4.1 Skill Cues

4.2 Basic Skills

4.3 Skill Sentences

4.4 Kinesiology

4.5 I'm Just Learning

For skill cue assessments 4.1 through 4.5 look for answers that are specific skill cues rather than general skill cues. For example, for the overhand throw "Step forward on the opposite foot as you throw" is a more specific answer than "Step forward." As stated in the rubric, if all skill cues are specific and correct, the assessment would earn a score of 3. If the cues are specific and the student did something extra to support his or her answers, the assessment would earn a score of 4.

Skill Cue Assessments With Added Creativity

4.6 Imagine That . . .

4.7 The Alien

4.8 Hey! I'm Talking to You!

4.9 Dear Mom, Dad, Grandma, or Grandpa

4.10 Teach Me!

4.11 Help Me! Tryouts Are Next Week!

4.12 Look Closely

4.13 Magical Sports Equipment

4.14 Picture It

4.15 You Ought to Be in Pictures!

4.16 Show Me What You Know—You Choose How!

Essentially, assessments 4.6 through 4.16 are asking students to identify the skill cues for the given skill. Within the assignment if the skill cues are correct and specific, the response would earn a score of 3. If the students went the extra mile and met the criteria on the rubric, the response would earn a score of 4.

Self-Assessments and Peer Assessments

4.17 Skill Stages—The answers for this self-assessment will depend on student performance. If you notice that a student is not accurate or not able to be objective, discuss the problem with him or her one on one.

4.18 Mechanics Check 1—The answers for this self-assessment will depend on student performance. If you notice that a student is not accurate or not able to be objective, discuss the problem with him or her one on one.

4.19 Mechanics Check 2—The answers for this peer assessment will depend on student performance. If you notice that a student is unable to be objective, discuss the problem with him or her one on one.

4.20 Accuracy Check—This assessment is based on accuracy of performance, and the score will depend on the student's performance.

Teacher Observation Tools

4.21 Assessing Student Performance—This teacher observation tool is used to record student performance.

4.22 Skill Stages—Teacher Assessment—This teacher observation tool is used to record student performance.

Skill-Tracking Assessments

4.23 Personal Best Skill Tracking

4.24 To 100!

4.25 Graduating Numbers

4.26 Time Trials

4.27 Group Challenge—Double It

4.28 Using Feedback to Improve Performance—The key to scoring this assessment is the student's ability to be specific about the physical changes that he or she needs to make to change the accuracy and consistency of the movement and whether this process brought about consistency in performance.

Assessment sheets 4.23 through 4.27 are skill-tracking assessments that allow students to track their improvement over time. What they accomplish will depend on performance.

Chapter 5: Concept Connection

5.1 Understanding Concepts—Apply It!—Answers will vary according to the skill and concepts targeted. Students need to make the connection between understanding the concepts and improving performance.

5.2 Understanding Concepts—Picture It!—Answers will vary according to the skill and concepts targeted. Students need to make the connection between understanding the concepts and improving performance through their illustrations and labels.

Application Assessments

5.3 Locomotor and Axial (Nonlocomotor) Movements

5.4 Using Space

5.5 Moving in Different Directions

5.6 Shapes—Narrow, Wide, Twisted, Round, Symmetrical, and Asymmetrical

5.7 Using Different Qualities of Time

5.8 Using Different Qualities of Force

5.9 Meet, Part, Lead, and Follow

5.10 Mirrors

5.11 Unison and Contrast

5.12 Concepts

5.13 Creating Games—The games developed by students in response to this assessment will depend on the skills that they are working with. You will have to observe each performance according to the specifics outlined on the rubric.

The sequences developed by students in response to assessments 5.3 through 5.12 will depend on the skills that they are working with. You will have to observe each performance according to the specifics outlined on the rubric.

Chapter 6: Focus on Fitness

Fitness Goal Setting, Planning, Testing, and Reflecting

6.1 Fitness Assessment—The key to scoring this assessment is not whether the student reached the fitness standards or reached his or her goals. The key is whether he or she showed fitness improvement in the items on the fitness assessment, analyzed the information correctly and completely, and offered specific information. You will see marked improvement in the student's ability to set realistic goals if you use this assessment over three or four years.

Fitness Quick Checks

6.2 Fitness Quick Check—Health—1. three of the following: cardiorespiratory endurance, flexibility, muscular strength, muscular endurance, body composition, 2. possible answers: stronger heart muscle, lower risk factors for heart disease, healthful weight, more energy, 3. possible answers: better posture, muscle tone, more energy, stronger, 4. possible answers: better posture, fewer injuries, less likely to have low back pain

6.3 Fitness Quick Check—Components—1. three of the following: cardiorespiratory endurance, flexibility, muscular strength, muscular endurance, body composition, 2. three of the following: power, speed, agility, balance, coordination, reaction time

6.4 Fitness Quick Check—Risk Factors—1. something that increases the likelihood of something happening, 2. lack of exercise, high stress levels, being overweight or obese, smoking tobacco

6.5 Fitness Quick Check—Cardio, Cardio, Cardio—1. possible answers: fitness of the heart and lungs, being able to exercise for long periods without getting tired, 2. at least 20 minutes, 3. three to five, 4. at a medium intensity, at your target heart rate, 5. your heart rate, 6. heart gets stronger, slower resting heart rate, greater stroke volume, longer time to rest

6.6 Fitness Quick Check—Heart Rate—1. person B, 2. Person B's heart rate would be lower because this person has a stronger heart muscle that can pump more blood with each beat. If it pumps more blood with each beat

it doesn't have to pump as many times to do the same amount of work.

6.7 Fitness Quick Check—Heart Disease—1. high blood pressure, atherosclerosis, 2. fat, 3. heart attack, 4. strong, 5. lower, 6. arteries, 7. risk

6.8 Fitness Quick Check—Warm-Up—1. possible answers: raises the heart rate slowly, prepares the body for exercise, slowly gets muscles working, 2. possible answers: slow locomotor movements, flexibility exercises, brisk walk, balance activity

6.9 Fitness Quick Check—Cool-Down—1. possible answers: gradually slows the heart rate, thus preventing blood from pooling in the legs, which can cause light-headedness, 2. possible answers: slow locomotor movements, flexibility exercises, brisk walk, balance activity, any movements slower than those that you were doing in the workout

6.10 Fitness Quick Check—Skill—1. five out of the six: power, speed, agility, balance, coordination, reaction time, 2. possible answers: As an athlete you could break down your sport into components and work to improve them so that you can improve performance; you can focus on the components that are important for success in your specific sport.

6.11 Fitness Quick Check—Vocabulary—1. B, 2. A, 3. C

6.12 Fitness Quick Check—Training—1. When you want to improve a certain part of fitness you must train specifically to do so. Example: Running will not improve muscular endurance of the abdominals, but it will improve cardiorespiratory endurance. 2. doing more than the body is used to doing so that you can improve that part of fitness, 3. slowly increasing the amount of work you do so that you can improve

Written Application Assessments

6.13 Apply Your Fitness Knowledge—Amazing Technology

6.14 Apply Your Fitness Knowledge—You Can Talk?

6.15 Apply Your Fitness Knowledge—Components

6.16 Apply Your Fitness Knowledge—Prescribe It

6.17 Apply Your Fitness Knowledge—Off-Season Training?

For the fitness application assessments 6.13 through 6.25, the answers will vary according to the activities that students are working with. The key to scoring these assessments is to pay close attention to the rubrics and look for complete, correct responses. Going a bit further by providing specific examples, more details, or artwork to support responses earns a score of 4 on all assessments.

Making Connections Outside the Classroom

You can use forms 6.26 and 6.27 as extra credit. These assessments will help you see whether students are making the connections between what they are learning in physical education and their fitness habits. Some students will be motivated to turn them in, and some will not.

Chapter 7: Make Time to Strategize

Written Assessments

Forms 7.1 through 7.5 assess the student's knowledge and understanding of strategies for different types of games. Scoring will depend on the student's ability to provide correct, complete, and specific answers based on what has been included in the teaching and learning activities.

Strategy Self-Assessments and Peer Assessments

For all the self-assessments and peer assessments (forms 7.6–7.12) responses will depend on student performance and the ability to be objective when doing the assessments.

Strategy Application Assessments

The application assessments in forms 7.14 and 7.15 require students to apply their knowledge of strategy to the type of game being played. Responses must make a clear connection between the plan and the strategies worked on during the teaching and learning activities. All the information provided must be complete and correct.

Chapter 9: Clipboard Closure and Processing Partners

You use the lists of open-ended statements during class and as part of class closure to check for understanding. Answers will vary, and students will build on them as you lead class discussions. The statements do not provide a formal assessment, but they will help you check for understanding.

Chapter 10: Force It

10.1 Force It—Processing Partner Statements—You use the lists of open-ended statements during class and as part of class closure to check for understanding. Answers will vary, and students will build on them as you lead class discussions. The statements do not provide a formal assessment, but they will help you check for understanding.

10.2 Force It—Mechanics Check—This peer assessment focuses on throwing mechanics. The answers will depend on student performance and the assessor's ability to be objective. If you have a student who is unable to be objective, discuss it with him or her one on one.

10.3 Force It—The Alien—Students should be able to include the skill cues for throwing within the response. The skill cues identified should be those that you have stressed during the unit. Within the assignment if the skill cues are correct and specific, the response will earn a score of 3. If the students did extra work and met the criteria on the rubric, the response will earn a score of 4.

10.4 Force It—Pictures—The response should include pictures representing the force concepts covered in the unit. Labels must support the illustrations and specify the ways in which the body is being used to produce force while throwing for distance.

Chapter 11: Fly, Birdie, Fly

11.1 Fly, Birdie, Fly—Processing Partner Statements—This list of open-ended statements is used during class and as part of class closure to check for understanding. Answers will vary, and students will build on them as you lead class discussions. The statements do not provide a formal assessment, but they will help you check for understanding.

11.2 Fly, Birdie, Fly—Personal Best Skill Tracking—This skill-tracking sheet will allow students to track their improvement over time. What they accomplish will depend on performance. Check with students as they work to be sure that they are progressing with the skills identified. Offer additional instruction for those who need it.

11.3 Fly, Birdie, Fly—Daily Checkout—The answers to these self-reflection assessments will depend on student performance and the student's ability to make an objective assessment of his or her class performance.

11.4 Fly, Birdie, Fly—Peer Assessment—Responses will depend on student performance and the ability to be objective when doing self-assessments and peer assessments.

11.5 Fly, Birdie, Fly—Strategize!—Students should be able to produce an accurate description of a game situation in which the best strategy would be to use each skill. Encourage students to choose to support answers with drawings that will help them with this assessment.

Chapter 12: Planning on Fitness

12.1 Planning on Fitness—Thinking About Skill-Related Fitness—1. coordinated, 2. agility, 3. speed, 4. force, 5. static, 6. balance, 7. standing broad jump, 8. direction, 9. coordination, 10. skill

12.2 Planning on Fitness—Daily Checkout—The answers to these self-reflection assessments will depend on student performance and the student's ability to make an objective assessment of his or her class performance.

12.3 Planning on Fitness—Components—1. three of the following: cardiorespiratory endurance, flexibility, muscular strength, muscular endurance, body composition, 2. three of the following: power, speed, agility, balance, coordination, reaction time

12.4 Planning on Fitness—Prescribe It—Because each student chooses an activity for this assessment, the answers will vary. Students must be able to identify two of the skill-related components specific to the activity chosen and then describe a related training activity for each.

About the Author

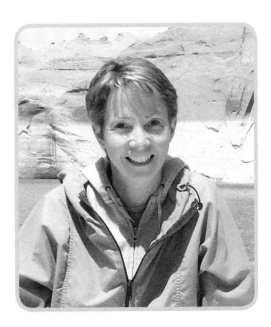

Liz Giles-Brown is currently a physical educator for grades K-8 at South Bristol School in South Bristol, Maine. In addition to having 17 years of experience teaching K-8 physical education, she has served as physical education curriculum chairperson and provided leadership in the assessment work done by her school union. Giles-Brown has also worked on state assessment development committees and currently serves on the expert review team for the Association for Supervision and Curriculum Development's (ASCD) Understanding by Design (UbD) online unit exchange.

Giles-Brown has also written two units that have been published on the Understanding by Design (UbD) Exchange and has presented numerous assessment workshops for her peers in the field of physical education. Giles-Brown is a member of the American Alliance for Health, Physical Education, Recreation and Dance (AAHPERD) and Maine Association for Health, Physical Education, Recreation and Dance (MAHPERD). In 2004 she received the Distinguished Leadership Award in physical education curriculum, teaching, and assessment from MAHPERD, which also named her Elementary Physical Education Teacher of the Year in 1995.

Giles-Brown holds a master's degree in physical education, curriculum, and instruction. She currently resides with her husband, Tim, and son, Chase, in West Boothbay Harbor, Maine, where she enjoys hiking, biking, boating, and skiing in her spare time.

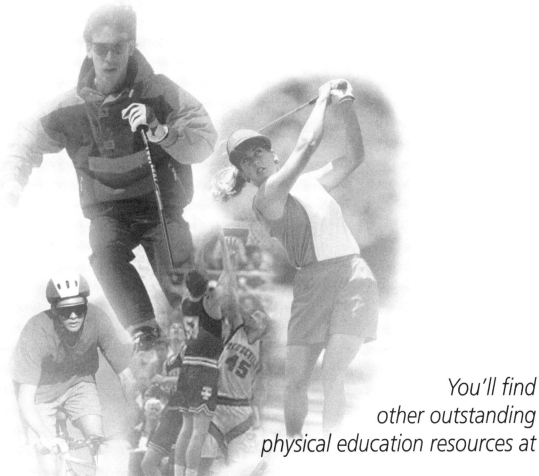

How to Use the CD-ROM

User instructions for *Physical Education Assessment Toolkit CD-ROM*

This CD-ROM contains

- More than 130 assessment forms used in the accompanying book. Each form is designed to be printed in black and white on letter-size paper.
- Nine full-color posters referenced in chapter 8 of the book. Each poster can be printed on letter-size paper or up to three times larger, to a maximum of 25.5 inches by 33 inches.

These resources are easy to pick and choose from and help you tailor your teaching to individual or local school needs. Just print them out and they're ready to use as is or customize for your specific plans. What's more, you can print the posters big enough to hang up in the classroom or small enough to hand out to students.

System Requirements

You can use this CD-ROM on either a Windows®-based PC or a Macintosh computer.

Windows

- IBM PC compatible with Pentium® processor
- Windows® 98/NT 4.0/2000/ME/XP
- Adobe Acrobat Reader®
- At least 16 MB RAM with 32 MB recommended
- 4x CD-ROM drive
- Inkjet or laser printer (optional)
- 256 colors
- Mouse

Macintosh

- Power Mac® recommended
- System 9.x or higher
- Adobe Acrobat Reader®
- At least 16 MB RAM with 32 MB recommended
- 4x CD-ROM drive
- Inkjet or laser printer (optional)
- 256 colors
- Mouse

User Instructions

Windows

1. Insert the *Physical Education Assessment Toolkit CD-ROM*. (*Note:* The CD-ROM must be present in the drive at all times.) The CD-ROM should launch automatically. If not, proceed to step 2.
2. Select the "My Computer" icon from the desktop.
3. Select the CD-ROM drive.
4. Open the "Launch.htm" file.
5. Follow the instructions on screen.

Macintosh

1. Insert the *Physical Education Assessment Toolkit CD-ROM*. (*Note:* The CD-ROM must be present in the drive at all times.)
2. Double-click the CD icon located on the desktop.
3. Open the "Start" file.
4. Follow the instructions on screen.

Note: OSX users, you must first open Acrobat Reader®, then select the file you wish to view from your CD-ROM drive and open the file from within Acrobat Reader®. For MacOS 10.1 and 10.2, you may need to be in Classic mode for the links on the table of contents to work correctly.

For product information or customer support:

E-mail: support@hkusa.com
Phone: 217-351-5076 (ext. 2970)
Fax: 217-351-2674
Web site: www.HumanKinetics.com